Proctology

PROCTOLOGY

Dr. Dale G. Keighley

International Academy of Proctology
American Osteopathic College of Proctology
East-Central States Osteopathic Society of Proctology
Clinical Professor of Proctology—
Ohio University College of Osteopathic Medicine

AN EXPOSITION-UNIVERSITY BOOK

Exposition Press   Hicksville, New York

CONTENTS

Contents

Contents

PREFACE

The purpose of this book is not to impress my proctological peers with my knowledge of didactic trivia, my skill as an artist, or my grammatical expertise. It is rather to give the average practitioner a better insight into the field of proctology and possibly to allow him to feel more comfortable doing a few rectal procedures in his office.

With many proctological thanks over the years to:

Dr. C. Charles Alexander
Dr. Harry Bacon
Dr. Gene Barbour
Dr. James Barron
Dr. John Bartizal
Dr. Edmund Bowman
Dr. Louis Buie
Dr. Alfred Cantor
Dr. Chester Chicky
Dr. Warren Cole
Dr. J. Joseph Cronin

Dr. Ralph Deger
Dr. George Dunk
Dr. Peter Eastman
Dr. Eugene Egle
Dr. Kenneth French
Dr. Arthur Friedman
Dr. Robert Gillon
Dr. Benjamin Gross
Dr. Harry Haltzman
Dr. Donald Hauck
Dr. Leo Hoersting

9

Dr. Louis Hoersting
Dr. Harold Kirsh
Dr. Joseph Lefler
Dr. LeRoy Lovelidge
Dr. Melumphy
Dr. Allan Miller
Dr. Thomas Miller
Dr. Carlton Noll
Dr. E. Duane Powers
Dr. Irving Schwartz
Dr. Richard Shackelford
Dr. Hiromi Shinya
Dr. Philip Slosberg

Dr. Ed Slowik
Dr. Julius Sobel
Dr. Leon Smeyne
Dr. Lee Smith
Dr. Frank Stanton
Dr. Lester Tavel
Dr. Ed Thorington
Dr. Robert Turell
Dr. Rudi Wadle
Dr. Earle Waters
Dr. George Waugh
Dr. Howard Weinstock
Dr. G. Zauder

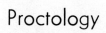

Proctology

PHYSIOLOGICAL ANATOMY 1

THE ASCENDING COLON is about 2½ times the diameter of the left colon. Here cancer is less likely to completely encircle the bowel. The most common lesions in this section occur at the junction of the cecum and the colon due to the larger caliber and the fluid fecal content.

The transverse colon lies more anteriorly and is therefore easier to palpate. Tumors here tend to invade contiguously the tail of the pancreas, the spleen, and the kidney.

The descending colon is smaller in caliber, weaker in peristaltic action, and poorer in blood supply. The function is storage prior to expulsion. The fecal content is more solid and not as easily propelled through a narrowed area of bowel. Lesions here usually tend to encircle the bowel and cause obstruction.

The rectum is rather large and relatively insensitive, allowing lesions in this area to attain great size before producing pain or causing obstruction. The ileocecal valve, when competent, allows the escape of all intestinal contents into the colon but no reverse flow from the cecum into the ileum.

13

BLOOD SUPPLY OF THE COLON AND RECTUM

Superior Mesenteric Artery

The *ileocolic artery* supplies the appendix, cecum, and lower ascending colon.
The *right colic artery* supplies the ascending colon.
The *middle colic artery* supplies hepatic flexure and the traverse colon.

Inferior Mesenteric Artery

The *left colic artery* supplies the descending colon.
The *sigmoidal arteries* supply the sigmoid colon.
The *superior hemorrhoidal artery* supplies the proximal rectum.

Internal Iliac Arteries

The *middle hemorrhoidal arteries* supply the middle rectum.
The *internal pudendal arteries* supply the distal rectum.
The *inferior hemorrhoidal arteries* supply the distal rectum.

The *lymphatics* of the colon consist of the *epicolic nodes, paracolic nodes, intermediate nodes*, and *principal nodes*. The lymphatics of the rectum are the intramural system, the intermediary system, and the extramural system. The mestastatic spread of a rectosigmoid carcinoma will most likely be to the periaortic nodes.

HEMORRHOIDAL PLEXUS

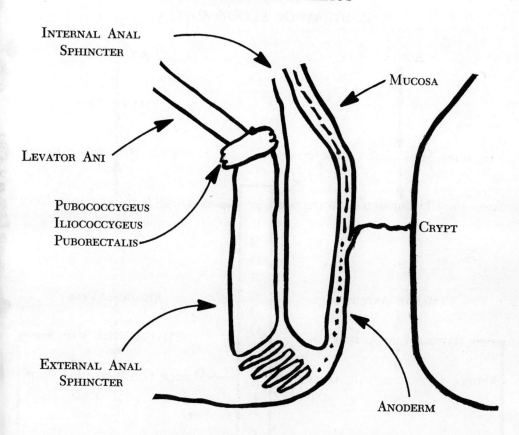

INTERNAL ANAL
SPHINCTER

MUCOSA

LEVATOR ANI

PUBOCOCCYGEUS
ILIOCOCCYGEUS
PUBORECTALIS

CRYPT

EXTERNAL ANAL
SPHINCTER

ANODERM

NOTE: *For simplification, the ischiococcygeus
and rectococcygeus are not shown on
drawing.*

DIAGRAM OF BLOOD SUPPLY

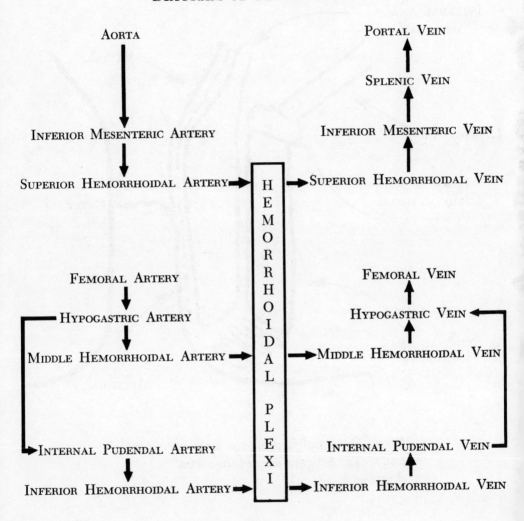

SYMPTOMS

2

PAIN

Increased with Stool

    Anal Fissure
    Anal Ulcer
    Stenosis

Constant

    Anal Ulcer
    Abrasion
    External Thrombotic Hemorrhoid
    External Clot
    Abscess
    Neoplasm
    Trauma
    Proctalgia Fugax
    Severe Pruritus Ani

17

Condylomata
Anal Fissure

Character

Sharp, Lancinating (Below anorectal line)
Constant Pressure (Above anorectal line)

I would like to preface this section by citing excerpts from a humorous account of a proctological patient. I am sure that most of us have seen this or similar efforts. Unfortunately so have many patients who have rectal symptomatology.

"Have you ever had hemorrhoids? Well, brother, if you have them, keep them. Don't let anybody get their hands on them. I offered mine to science and that was my first mistake. . . . The night before surgery, several deceptive practices take place. First, as a touch of indoctrination and toughening up, the rear end and surrounding terrain are shaven—dry, not wet. Try it on a day's growth of beard. . . . New blades don't count, the older they are the better. . . . Even the four-foot needle used for the anesthetic, etc. . . .

"A little while later it hits you so hard you can't breathe . . . hot, soaring pains in solid waves permeate your rear and hit every nerve in your body. . . . They left a red-hot iron in you or at least a pint of molten lead. You can't escape it. Every odd second your muscles pull in a spasmodic, contracting spasm. . . . Even a couple of morphine shots only dull it slightly."

And then the author's coup de grace: "The last part of this first movement and next ten or twelve more were a constant passing of broken bottles, old razor blades, molten lead, and sulfuric acid nicely garnished with bits of barbed wire, porcupine quills, and jagged pieces of other ingredients such as tin cans."

This glowing account of the pain associated with proctological

18

procedures is certainly enough to deter many patients from presenting themselves to a physician for examination in regard to a rectal complaint.

The symptom of rectal pain is responsible for more deaths than any other proctological symptom. This is due to the fact that rectal pain results in the lack of differential diagnosis in several ways.

First, rectal pain is often believed by the general public as being due to hemorrhoids alone. These patients fear the legendary pain associated with rectal examination. Consequently, many are attracted by advertisements of diverse popular proprietary products in all advertising media promising painless rectal cures, often showing 20cc. syringes with 10-gauge trochars as an indication of the negative psychological aspects of the surgical procedures.

The advertisements often indicate that the magic compound "shrinks hemorrhoids." Of course, when an external thrombotic hemorrhoid resolves in five to seven days, the patient must assume that this was the direct result of the proprietary product rather than the benevolence of Mother Nature. Few of these companies direct the patient to consult a physician if symptoms persist. As a tragic consequence, the patient with rectal pain often delays the definitive diagnosis of the etiology of the rectal pain, thereby resulting in a malignant head start that no physician can adequately treat.

Second, there is the physician who has no respect for the density of pain sensors of the anorectal area and uses his finger as a battering ram as if in a hurry to relieve his finger of aching arthritis with the intrarectal warmth of the patient. These men, of course, unnecessarily cause the pain which the patient relates to his friends and thereby instills in them the fear that results in their refusal to appear for needed, indicated, definitive examination.

Responsible for a successful proctosigmoidoscopic examination is the manner in which the initial examining finger is inserted into the patient's anorectal orifice. It must be held against the longitudinal axis of the anal slit with mild pressure until the anal sphincter relaxes around the finger. This gentle approach follows with any instrumentation. I further do not believe that a 19mm.-diameter sigmoidoscope is necessary in most cases. I use a 15mm. fiber optic sigmoidoscope and find it much more acceptable to the patient and certainly satisfactory for screening purposes.

I also feel that the patient must be adequately informed by the proctologist exactly what pathology is present and what, generally, is going to be done to correct the situation. Fear is the greatest single problem in the proctological patient. A scared patient is a tense patient and a tense patient is going to have more painful spincter spasm. In my office we use a twelve-page pamphlet outlining in as much detail as feasible what the patient is to expect during the examination as well as during the pre- and post-op periods.

It is my opinion that many patients complain not of the pain that they are currently having but of the pain that they feel they will be forced to endure in the immediate future. These factors are extremely important and vital, because, as proctologists, we are strangers to the patient and do not have the trust that the patient has in his family doctor. We must earn this trust with gentleness and understanding.

Third, we come to the pain of the postoperative period—the aforementioned broken glass and red-hot razor blades—which has kept many a soul from presenting himself for definitive diagnosis for fear of possible ensuing surgery.

It becomes evident that it behooves us to do all in our power to minimize this form of "Bard-Parker" poisoning. As has previously been mentioned, we must consider in this endeavor the preoperative, and postoperative periods.

Before surgery the physician must employ gentleness at all times in examining the patient and utilize vocal reassurance as well as proper informative rapport. Many things can be done at the surgical table to minimize postoperative pain. There must be a respect for tissue, with judicious dissection as indicated and governed by the pathology present in each case.

Today, most hemorrhoids may be treated by the rubber-band technique. This technique, with its minimal discomfort and disability to the patient, should be utilized as often as possible.

It is of paramount importance to use as little suture as absolutely necessary below the anorectal line.

If you use an electrosurgical technique remember that you are using the modality to excise and fulgerate pathological tissue, not to barbecue the entire rear half of the patient.

Because spasm of the sphincter may initiate or increase pain, the fibers of the sphincter are partially bisected by many men.

I infiltrate the anal region at surgery with a solution composed of seven centimeters of xylocaine with epinephrine. I feel this is helpful by decreasing bleeding due to the vasoconstrictive effect of the epinephrine, thereby decreasing the amount of suture and/or cautery used.

I know that some men use a long-acting, oil-soluble anesthetic at surgery. Some feel that this affords great aid in controlling postoperative pain. I have never personally done this, because of a morbid fear of the possibility of slough, but as a great proctologist, Dr. Alfred Cantor, once quoted, "There are many roads to Rome."

After surgery we must understand the concept that pain is a very personal thing. What is painful to one individual may not bother another, but, as far as the first individual is concerned, the pain is real and must be treated as such. Pain has two components, *perception* and *reaction*. The *perception* of pain is a purely physiological mechanism and depends on the interactions of nerve endings and conduction pathways. The *reaction* to pain is basically psychogenic, highly individualized, and modified by complex functions and factors. The interpretation of pain is dependent on the degree of stimulus, the type of tissue receiving the stimulus, and the patient's threshold.

Another concept in which I firmly believe is that, if pain is not treated at its outset, because of a pain-fear-pain vicious cycle, more analgesic is required to bring it under control. I feel that there is no excuse for a patient to have severe pain in a hospital situation.

Having stated my basic concepts concerning pain I would like to discuss my postoperative pain control measures:

Demerol 100mg. Q. 3-4 hrs. prn, on the day of surgery and the first postoperative day.

Fiorinal #3 Q. 3-4 hrs. prn, thereafter.

Sitz baths T.I.D. $\times$ 10 minutes beginning on the second postoperative day to get rid of the morning stiffness of the postoperative anorectal region. I have tried heat pads, hydrothermic pads, and diathermy, but still prefer the sitz bath. The point must be made to the floor nurses that the morning sitz bath is of paramount importance.

An ice bag to the area on the day of surgery, and first postoperative day, followed by a warm water bottle thereafter.

Diothane cream and ARD pads for patient application.

Tucks for cleanliness.

Most important is a routine order stating that, if the pain medication does not relieve the patient's pain, I am to be notified, night or day. This is to abolish the "Clara Barton" of the night shift from telling one of my patients that "they can't have anything for pain for another hour—and it's all in their head anyway." That tells you what she knows about anatomy.

Symptoms

BLEEDING

N.B.: TRANSANAL BLEEDING IS CARCINOMA UNTIL PROVEN OTHERWISE.

Color

> Dark   (Upper Gastrointestinal)
> Bright (Lower Gastrointestinal)
> (Even though the color really depends on transit rate through the colon)

Location

> Mixed with stool   (Lesions of right colon)
> After stool   (Lesions of lower colon or rectum)

With Anorectal Pain (Lesion below the anorectal line)

> Fissure
> Hemorrhoids
> Proctitis
> Cryptitis
> Draining Abscess
> Anal Neoplasm
> Anal Ulcer
> Fungal Lesions
> Dermatological Excoriations
> Condylomata

Without Anorectal Pain (Often in malignancies)

> Internal Hemorrhoids
> Proctitis

Neoplasm
Ulcerative Colitis
Crohn's Disease
Meckel's Diverticulum
Diverticulitis
Intussusception
Lesion of the upper GI tract
Systemic disease

N.B.: 1. The color of the blood depends on the motility of the gut. Do not use this as an indication of what level the blood is coming from.

        2. The amount of blood is not related to the degree of pathology.

PROTRUSION
(or Swelling)

With Pain

    Abscess
    Thrombotic Hemorrhoid
    Sentinal Pile
    Neoplasm
    Condylomata

Without Pain

    Prolapsed Internal Hemorrhoids (unless strangulated)

Prolapsed Hypertrophied Papilla
Skin Tag

CHANGE IN BOWEL HABIT

Constipation

Decreased Defecation Reflex (due to chronic stretching of rectal vault from neglect of reflex)
Debilitating Diseases
Gastric Carcinoma
Bowel Spasm
Obstructed Lumen
Sphincter spasm (due to painful anal lesions)

Narrow Stools

Malignancy
Stenosis

Diarrhea

Colonic Ulceration
Colonic Inflammation
Mesenteric Ischemia
Overjudicious Use of Antibiotics
Lactose Deficiency
Malabsorption Syndrome
Neoplastic Disease
Achlorhydria

Impaction (liquid stool escaping around large mass)
Incontinent Sphincter

Alternating Diarrhea and Constipation

Colitis
Polyposis
Malignancy
Diverticulitis

Night Stools

Occasionally Neoplastic Disease

Constipation

Etiology

Cortical Inhibition
Poor bowel habits due to neglect of reflex
Wasting Diseases
Decreases the "pushing power"
Decreased Gastric Motility
Gastro-colic reflex decreased in gastric carcinoma
Bowel Spasm
Due to local inflamation
Lumenal Obstruction
Due to neoplasm
Sphincter Spasm
Due to acute proctitis, fissure, etc.
Dilated Rectal vault
Due to constipatory storage (poor bowel habits) decreasing the defecation reflex

TREATMENT

1. The patient should not ignore the urge to defecate (preferably at definite regular time).

2. The patient should adhere to a nutritionally balanced diet (including fruits and vegetables) at regular intervals.

3. There should be an adequate fluid intake (six glasses of water per day).

4. Mild morning exercise is beneficial.

5. Digital breakup and partial removal of impaction if present followed in an adult patient with two Dulcolax tablets.

6. The underlying cause must be determined, utilizing the list of etiologies and specific therapy instituted.

Diarrhea

CLASSIFICATION

Osmotic Diarrhea—Stops when oral intake is stopped

1. Laxatives

2. Surgery (stomach, intestines)

3. Malabsorption syndromes
    a. Fat
    b. Glucose—Galactose

4. Enzyme deficiency (disaccharidase)

5. Immune deficiency
   a. IgA Deficiency
   b. Lymphonodular hyperplasias

6. Infections

7. Defective mucosal permeability resulting in excess bile acids or hydroxy—fatty acids in colon
   a. Crohn's disease
   b. Ileal resection

8. Defective active transport (chloride, hexose)

9. Heavy metal ingestion (copper, tin, zinc)

Secretory Diarrhea—Persists after oral intake is stopped

1. Infections

2. Infestations

3. Humoral Agents
   a. Vaso-active intestinal polypeptide
   b. Zollinger-Ellison syndrome
   c. Thyroid cancer

4. Excess bile acids or hydroxy—fatty acids in colon

5. Sprue

6. Ulcerative colitis

7. Intestinal obstruction

8. Tumors of colon

Acute Diarrheas

1. With Bleeding

    a. Causative agent not demonstrable
        Ischemic colitis
        Pseudomembranous colitis
        Acute stage of chronic ulcerative colitis
        Diverticulitis
        Vasculitis of colon
    b. Causative agent demonstrable
        Amebiasis
        Shigella
        Salmonella

2. Without Bleeding
    a. Organism not cultured in stool
        Acute gastroenteritis (viral)
        Food poisoning
        Antibiotic induced
    b. Agent cultured
        Salmonella
        Pathologic E. Coli
        Cholera

DISCHARGE

Pus

    Fistula
    Abscess
    Ulcerative Colitis

Mucous

    Internal Hemorrhoids
    Proctitis

Malignancy
Indicates Irritation of Mucosa
Ulcerative Colitis
Nonulcerative Colitis

Serous

Pruritus Ani
Condylomata Accuminata
Fungi

PRURITUS ANI
(Itching)

Pruritus ani is an intractable perianal itching characterized by periods of remission and recurrence and accompanied by an alteration in the epidermis of the region due to irritation of the peripheral nerve endings. This is caused by local or systemic disease. The pain is variable depending on the tolerance of the individual patient. This problem is more prevalent in males than in females by 50%. It is also greater between the ages of 20 to 45 and is greater in sedentary occupations. Approximately 10 to 25% of the adult population is plagued with this malady.

There are several factors involved in the occurrence of pruritus ani. There is no universal etiological agent, nor is there a universal therapy. The skin in the anal region is more alkaline than elsewhere in the body. The secretions of the glands in the area are controlled in part by the emotional stress of the individual. The anal areas most susceptible to pruritus are one inch around the anus and also an area one to two inches in length and one inch wide just anterior to the anus.

Pruritus ani is worse at night. The more the person scratches, the worse the itch becomes. The patient will continue to scratch no matter how well he is convinced that this will make the condition worse.

The skin is thickened, there is an increase in pigmentation, and fissures or excoriations are common. The anal skin folds are increased in size. The skin may be reddish-blue from underlying inflammation, white, moist and macerated, or dry and scaling.

The etiologies of pruritus ani are primary and secondary. The primary, or idiopathic causes, are responsible for about 45% of all pruritus ani and are termed by some writers neurodermatitis. This is the anxiety-inch-anxiety-itch syndrome that is so difficult for the practitioner to cope with. The itching in these patients seems to be increased to worry, fright, and overwork. Some authors have associated this with premature ejaculation in males, frigidity in females, the uncertainty of the male as to his sex, and in others as an analogue of masturbation.

The secondary causes of pruritus ani are subdivided into dermatologic, systemic, and surgical divisions. Dermatological lesions are responsible for about 20% of pruritus ani. These are usually abetted by poor hygiene. These may be associated with skin disease, allergy, infections, fungus, parasites, rare lesions, or diet.

Skin Disease

> Psoriasis
> Seborrheic Dermatitis
> Atrophic Eczema
> Lichen Planus
> Lichen Sclerosis Et Atrophicus

Allergy

    Anesthetics
    Antihistamines
    Soap and Detergents
    Clothing
    Toilet Paper Dye (especially yellow)
    Antibiotics
    Other Medications (Quinine, Morphine, Belladonna)
    Ad Nauseam

Infections and Fungus

    Monilia
    Dermatophytosis
    Trichomonas
    Bacteria

Parasites

    Scabies
    Pinworms
    Amebiasis
    Pediculosis
    Creeping Eruption

Rare Lesions

    Extramammary Paget's Disease
    Giant Comedomes

Diet

    Gormandizing
    Highly Seasoned Foods
    Condiments

Tomatoes
Berries
Beer
Chronic Alcoholism
Chocolate
Shellfish
Bran
Cheese
Nuts
Coffee
Tea
Cola
Alcohol

Systemic diseases are responsible for about 10% of pruritus ani. A partial list of systemic etiologies follows:

Liver Disease—Portal Congestion
Lymphoma
Polycythemia Vera
Vitamin A and B Deficiency
Nephritis
Uremia
Gall Bladder Disease
Subclinical Jaundice
Gastrointestinal Disease
Gout (Acidosis)
Rheumatism
Lues
Tuberculosis

Vasomotor Imbalance
Endocrinological Problems
    Hypoadrenia
    Diabetes (Monilia)
    Hypopituitarism
    Senility
    Obesity
    Altered Cholesterols

Surgical causes account for about 25% of pruritus ani.

Rectal

    Fissures
    Fistulae
    Hemorrhoids
    Draining Sinuses
    Anal Ulcers
    Rectal Prolapse
    Papillitis
    Previous Surgery
    Venous Stasis
    Cryptitis
    Skin Tags
    Neoplasms
    Strictures
    Foreign Bodies
    Fecal Impaction
    Passage of Hard Stools

Uterus

    Displacement

Inflammation
Pregnancy
Tumors
Procidentia

Ovary

Cysts
Tumors

Prostate

Hypertrophy
Inflammation
Tumors

Bladder

Inflammation
Tumors
Lithiasis

Urethra

Stricture
Phimosis
Inflammation

It should be obvious after the foregoing material that effective therapy of pruritus ani must include general hygienic measures and local treatment aimed at eradicating the symptomatology, followed by determination of the etiological agent or agents. Then and only then may specific therapeusis be instituted. It is well to adhere to a regime that will halt the progress of the pruritus until the causative factor is uncovered. The therapeutic modalities are legion. Several of the more frequent treatments follow:

Proctology

1. Stop all medications.

2. Use Burrow's solution compresses.

3. Use cool tap water sitz baths.

4. Avoid tight clothing.

5. Use steroid creams—better than radiation (Grenz Rays).

6. Use steroids if very severe.

7. Tell patient to decrease scratching, not stop completely.

8. Use vitamin therapy.

9. Avoid sensitizing drugs.

10. Scrub with soap during bathing.

11. Stop toilet paper. Use moistened cotton Tucks.

12. If skin is dry and scaly, add coal tar to steroid cream.

13. No opiates.

14. No alcohol.

15. Decrease smoking.

16. No condiments or peppery foods.

17. Tranquilizers.

18. Temaril.

19. Trim fingernails short.

20. Use psychiatric therapy if indicated.

21. Use white toilet paper only (yellow worst).

22. Use camphor-phenol solution.

23. Cryo application on 4 quadrants of the anus (in intractable cases).

24. Corn starch (during daytime).

25. Corticaine cream.

26. Minute injection of ethanol subcutaneously in a gridwork pattern. (This, however, often results in an undesirable tissue slough.)

27. Ball's Operation (which is a cloverleaf subcutaneous neurotomy).

About 50% of the cases of pruritus ani defy determination of their etiologies and are nonresponsive to medical therapeutic regime. To cope with these cases, techniques have evolved which interrupt the peripheral nerve endings by either chemical means or surgical undercutting procedures known as neurotomies, such as number 23, number 26, and number 27.

28. Change the pH of the stool with Acidulin.

29. Avoid chocolate, beer, tomatoes, coffee, tea.

METHODS OF EXAMINATION 3

PROCTOSIGMOIDOSCOPY

A SATISFACTORY EXAMINATION of the lower end of the digestive tract is essential for the early diagnosis of pathology of this region. This examination should be performed by the general practioner just as are cancer smears of the cervix. The purpose of the following is to equip the general practitioner with the basic knowledge involved in a comprehensive examination of the anorectum.

The best position for proctosigmoidoscopy is on a Ritter-type table in a knee-chest position. These tables are quite expensive. An alternative position is the Sim's position, in which the patient is placed in a left lateral position with the lower leg straight and the upper leg flexed in a knee-chest position and the perianal region is visually inspected for:

Discharge
Protrusions

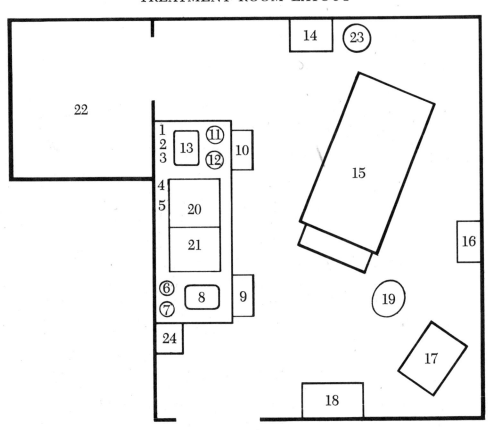

1. Hydrogen peroxide
2. Camphor/Phenol solution (50% of each)
3. Trichloracetic acid
4. Cellucotton wipes cut from roll to $4'' \times 5''$
5. Mercresin spray
6. $3'' \times 3''$ sponges
7. Applicator sticks
8. Instrument boat
9. Ligator sets (loaded) in drawer
10. Sigmoidoscopes in drawer
11. K-Y jelly in jar
12. Americaine in jar (20% Benzocaine)
13. Plastic anoscopes
14. Suction unit with table sheets on top
15. Ritter table
16. Bovie unit
17. Chair
18. Drawer with local, syringes, blades, and suture
19. Light
20. Sink for dirty instruments
21. Sink for washing instruments
22. Bath
23. Cryosurgical unit
24. Trash

Ulcerations
Sinuses
Fissure
Pinworms
Patulous sphincter
Discolorations
Edema
Evidence of trauma
Sentinal pile
Prolapsed structures
Condylomata
Abscess
Hypertrophied skin folds
Skin tags
Excoriations
Fistulous openings
Blood

The digital examination should follow vocal reassurance to the patient. The gloved, well-lubricated index finger is gently inserted into the anus. The finger should be held with firmness against the external sphincter until that muscle is felt to relax. The lateral surfaces of the examining finger should be anterior-posterior in direction, because this more nearly approximates the natural curvature of the anal slit. The examiner should be aware of:

Sphincter tone
Thrombosed internal hemorrhoids
Impacted feces
Areas of pain

Soft, fluctuant tender abscess areas
Anal fissure
Fistulae
Polyps
Stricture
Hypertrophied anal papillae
Firm annular lesions (malignancies)
Condylomata
Tumors
Foreign bodies
Contiguous structures (uterus, prostate, Blummer's shelf lesions)

N.B.: Internal hemorrhoids are not palpable unless they are thrombosed.

This digital examination should be followed with a procto-sigmoidoscopic examination. (The patient should have an enema two hours before the examination.) This portion of the examination is very important, because 45% of the population above the age of 40 years has anorectal pathology that needs treatment. The following pathologies may be noted with this procedure:

Bleeding Points
Ulcerations
Polyps
Diverticuli
Melanosis Coli
Inflammation
Hypertrophied Papillae
Fissure En Ano

Petecchiae
Cryptitis
Discharges (Blood, Pus, Mucous)
Neoplasms
Condylomata
Papillitis
Hemorrhoids
Mucosal Redundancy

The successful proctosigmoidoscopic examination is marked with gentleness and reassurance to the patient. It is best to keep the instruments under cover until the patient is positioned. The lubricated anoscope is inserted to examine the hemorrhoidal area and to divulge the anus gently. The sigmoidoscope is then well lubricated and inserted slowly into the anal canal with firm, steady pressure for about two inches, pointing the instrument to the patient's navel. The scope is then directed to the hollow of the sacrum and the obturator is then removed. Some important points in sigmoidoscopy follow:

1. Never advance the scope unless the lumen is clearly visible directly ahead.

2. Do not feel that you must pass the instrument "to the hilt" on every patient.

3. If you meet with difficulty or obstruction, stop at that level.

4. If you want, you may insufflate air into the scope to balloon out the mucosa. This will result in cramping for the patient, which will pass when you open up the lens and allow the air to pass out.

5. If you press the instrument against bowel wall instead of lumen, the mucosa will blanche and the patient will complain of sharp pain.

6. Always advance the scope slowly and only if the lumen is visible.

7. Some normal structures which will be present are:

   a. The Semilunar Valves of Houston
   Inferior (Left Posterior): 3.2″ above the anal verge
   Middle (Right Anterior): 4.4″ above the anal verge
   Superior (Left Posterior): 5″ above the anal verge
   b. The Recto-Sigmoid Junction (6.5-7.5″ above the anal verge).
   At the region the lumen no longer appears round but appears to be a wormy (wavy) slit
   c. The pulsations of the left hypogastric artery may be visible in the sigmoid.

I feel that at this time the finest sigmoidoscopes are the Welch-Allen fiberoptic scopes. These come in several diameters (19mm., 15mm., and 11mm.). The 15mm. scope is the easiest to use and much less uncomfortable for the patient.

The disposable anoscope with obturator is an excellent anoscope for general office use and may be used for ligating hemorrhoids.

Being aware of and adhering to the several above-mentioned cautions, you are now ready to proceed with sigmoidoscopy by usage. The first few times you may reach only 15 to 16 centimeters depth. Do not be discouraged—the next time you may pass the instrument the entire 25 centimeters. Remember that even those of us who have passed the sigmoidoscope thousands of times occasionally do not reach 25 centimeters. At 15 centimeters depth you have examined deeper than many of your colleagues attempt to examine. This examination should give the practitioner pride in that he has done the patient a great service in a thorough exploration of the rectosigmoid.

COLONOSCOPY

The development of colonoscopy has added to our armamentarium one of the finest weapons against colonic cancer since the beginning of time. Through this instrument it is possible to directly examine the entire colonic mucosa, to biopsy suspected lesions, to obtain cytological specimens, and to remove pedunculated polyps. Various studies have indicated that 30% to 40% of neoplastic lesions may be missed by barium enema studies and diagnosed with a colonoscope in experienced hands.

I feel that the day is long gone when a physician may learn to perform colonoscopy without some formal training. It is extremely difficult to master the "slide techniques" without direct coaching to indicate the parameters of normal distension utilizing a teaching colonoscope attachment. I do want to include some pointers for the tyro colonoscopist, however, in order to keep the colonic perforation rate down to an acceptable one or two out of a thousand colonoscopies.

I find that most perforations occur in two areas. The most prevalent perforation is at a thin-walled diverticulum, especially in the geriatric patient. This problem is usually resultant from the overuse of air insufflation and the failure to decompress the bowel with light suction when extricating the colonoscope.

The second most common perforation suprisingly occurs at the peritoneal reflexion of the lower sigmoid colon where the bowel is fixed in position. This perforation, due to its location, presents marked problems in repair. This perforation at the peritoneal reflexion is due to the stretching of the bowel caused by the semicoil of the colonoscope. This is usually resultant from the injudicious usage of the slide technique in misinterpreting the springy rebound feeling with lessened advancement of the colonoscopic tip as observed by the colonoscopist.

I believe the following considerations should be observed in colonoscopic procedures:

1. Insufflation should be used as sparingly as possible, especially in the geriatric patient.

2. The colon should be decompressed with the use of suction on removal of the colonoscope.

3. It is my belief that the only polyps in which polypectomy should be attempted through the colonoscope should be polyps with a pedicular diameter of less than 0.5cm. This, of course, rules out the extraction of sessile polyps transcolonoscopically.

4. In utilizing the slide technique in passing the colonoscope, I feel that it is necessary in order to correlate the visual perception of the advancement with the inherent springlike resistance of the colonoscope that the colonoscopist should be the one who is actually inserting the scope.

5. In contrast to many of my fellow colonoscopists, I feel that the alpha maneuver is a dangerous procedure in which the potential problems greatly supersede the advantages. This is best demonstrated by flexing the tip of the colonoscope when it is out of the patient and rotating it 180 degrees; it is obvious that this can

inflict considerable trauma to abdominal viscera. If one would complicate this problem with an additional curve in the length of the scope and then rotate the scope 180 degrees, it is obvious that the potential trauma would be greatly compounded.

6. The colonic wall must constantly be observed for evidence of blanching, which would indicate exorbitant stretching of the bowel wall.

Remember:

Transanal bleeding is carcinoma until proven otherwise.

Preparation

To ensure a successful examination, it is important that the patient's entire colon be thoroughly clean. Low enemas, as used for proctologic preparation, are usually insufficient.

The following instructions are therefore recommended unless medically contraindicated:

1. Patient to have clear liquid diet only, on day preceding examination.

2. Dulcolax tabs, 2 at bedtime on the night before the examination (adult dose).

3. Nothing to eat or drink after bedtime until examination completed.

4. On the morning of the examination, *high* colonic enemas until clear. Patient should lie on left side until about one pint of warm, soapy water has run in slowly. Patient should then turn on back and more water introduced. Finally, patient should turn on right side until he/she cannot hold any more. Most people can hold better than one quart. Then evacuate. Repeat until clear return. This may require 2, 3, or 4 enemas.

HEMORRHOIDAL DISEASE 4

ENLARGED HEMORRHOIDAL VEINS are caused by anything that increases venous pressure on the hemorrhoidal plexus such as:

Erect human posture
Constipation
Diarrhea
Pregnancy
Lifting (including weight lifting)
Straining at stool
Coughing
Sneezing
Liver disease

PROGRESSION OF HEMORRHOIDAL DISEASE

The hemorrhoidal veins lie in loose connective tissue, and therefore their distension occurs easily from the above-mentioned factors. As the hemorrhoids distend they cause a separation of the mucosa from the muscularis layer, allowing for further engorgement of the venous plexus. This engorgement can reach a maximum, and at that point the venous plexus may rupture and a quantity of blood may be pushed into the anoderm, resulting in an "external hemorrhoid." This external hemorrhoid (clot) will absorb in 5 to 7 days, resulting in a skin tag.

The congested tissue of an engorged venous plexus results in a diminished blood flow in the area, which, as in any other part of the body, leads to inflamed tissue. In this area that inflammation is called proctitis. Proctitis may proceed into the crypts and crypt glands. This is called cryptitis. In some persons this infection may burrow from the crypt area through the surrounding tissues as a tract called a fistula to an abscess area.

This inflamed tissue area (proctitis) also may allow a tear to occur in the anal area. This tear is a fissure. This fissure, if of long standing, may have some tissues bunched up at its outer limit, which is called a "sentinel tag" of Brodie.

PROGRESSION OF HEMORRHOIDAL DISEASE

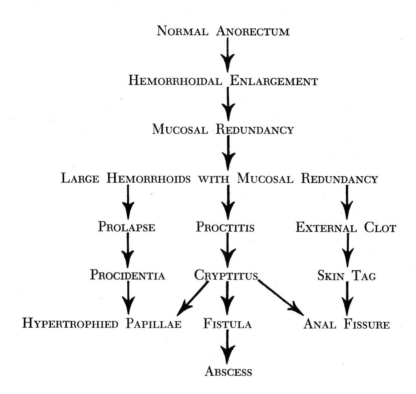

NORMAL ANORECTUM

HEMORRHOIDAL ENLARGEMENT

MUCOSAL REDUNDANCY

LARGE HEMORRHOIDS WITH MUCOSAL REDUNDANCY

PROLAPSE   PROCTITIS   EXTERNAL CLOT

PROCIDENTIA   CRYPTITUS   SKIN TAG

HYPERTROPHIED PAPILLAE   FISTULA   ANAL FISSURE

ABSCESS

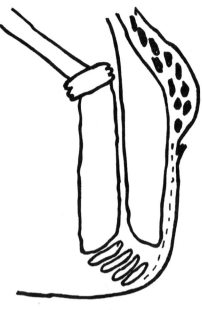

ENLARGED INTERNAL
HEMORRHOID

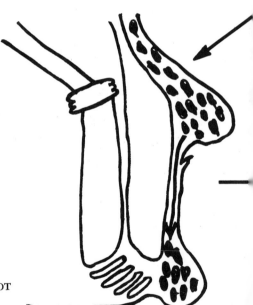

EXTERNAL CLOT

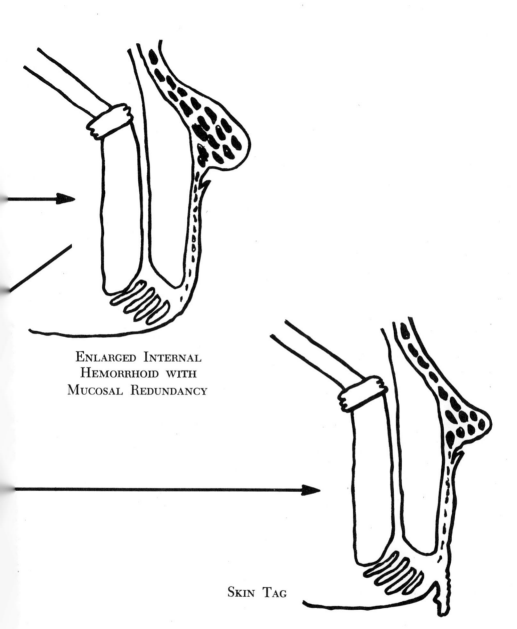

ENLARGED INTERNAL
HEMORRHOID WITH
MUCOSAL REDUNDANCY

SKIN TAG

PROCEDURES FOR INTERNAL HEMORRHOIDECTOMY 5

THE PROCEDURES for hemorrhoidectomy over the centuries have been extremely varied. I once heard Dr. Alfred Cantor state that "there are many roads to Rome" in this procedure. That is to say, if a physician has good results with one of the varied procedures, that procedure may be best for him. The problem is that if he does not try different techniques he can not appraise his results relative to other techniques. A few of the techniques are:

1. Ligation
2. Injection of a sclerosing solution
3. Cauterization (clamp and cautery)
4. Sharp radial dissection (clamp and suture)
5. Cryosurgery
6. Tube resection (Modified Whitehead)
7. Extreme dilation
8. Laser removal

LIGATION

The ligation treatment of hemorrhoids has existed for centuries. Nearly all cases of internal hemorrhoids can be treated by this technique, which offers the following advantages:

To the Doctor

1. It is a simple, quick office procedure.
2. No anesthetic is required (general or local).
3. No preparation is required.

To the Patient

1. No hospitalization is needed.
2. Postoperative urinary retention is extremely rare.
3. Postoperative bleeding of any consequence is extremely rare.
4. There is seldom a disablement from normal activities.
5. There is only minimal discomfort.

Several years ago I designed the Keighley ligator, which has several advantages over the other ligator sets:

1. less expensive
2. only an 8-inch shaft, making the procedure less cumbersome
3. all stainless steel
4. simple, one-piece construction
5. triggers with a positive pressure on the mucosa, resulting in a better seating of the band

This instrument is available from:

The Keighley Proctological Instrument Company
359 Forest Avenue
Dayton, Ohio 45405

The banding of hemorrhoids is more acceptable to the patient than hospital surgical procedures and therefore has resulted in a much larger proctological practice for the physicians utilizing this procedure. This technique should be used only on internal hemorrhoids, that is, hemorrhoidal masses above the junction of mucosa and anoderm. This junction (roughly at the level of the anal crypts) is known as the anorectal line. The mucosa above this line has no cutaneous pain fibers and may be cut, tied, or burned with only a resultant sensation of pressure. It is this physiological fact that allows the ligation of internal hemorrhoids with a minimum of patient discomfort.

The bands accomplish three things:

1. excise the hemorrhoidal plexus

2. remove the redundant mucosa

3. form a scar "tack" to adhere the mucosa to the muscularis

LOADING THE LIGATOR

A single band is pushed into the loading cone from the pointed end to about ⅛″ from the largest end of the cone. The loading cone is then inserted into the extended small cylinder of the ligator,

59

and then, with one brisk push by the fingers of the left hand, the band is transferred from the large end of the loading cone onto the extended small cylinder of the ligator as the ligator is held in the right hand. The ligator then may be triggered by squeezing the handles apart.

PROCEDURE

A well-lubricated medium-size anal speculum (the disposable plastic anoscopes serve very well) is inserted into the anal verge without local or general anesthetic. The internal hemorrhoids are observed usually at the right anterior, right posterior, and left lateral quadrants. The grasping forceps (passed through the cylinder of the loaded ligator) are used to grasp the body of the internal hemorrhoid, about 0.5cm. above the crypt line, and pull it into the double cylinder of the ligator. (At this point the patient should experience only a feeling of pressure. If the patient complains of sharp pain, the hemorrhoidal mass should be grasped at a slightly higher level.)

The ligator is then triggered, causing the small band to encircle the hemorrhoidal mass. The patient will usually have, as stated, a sensation of pressure, which will last about 20 hours. If desired, a mild analgesic will abate this pressure sensation. It is generally wise to have the patient on a stool softener during the period of ligation therapy. This procedure is repeated at weekly intervals on one hemorrhoidal mass per visit for three weeks, and then a follow up visit is recommended one or two weeks later.

Anal skin tags, if present and a bother to the patient, may be excised in the office under local anesthesia. If this is necessary hemostasis may be obtained by electrocoagulation.

HEMORRHOIDAL LIGATION

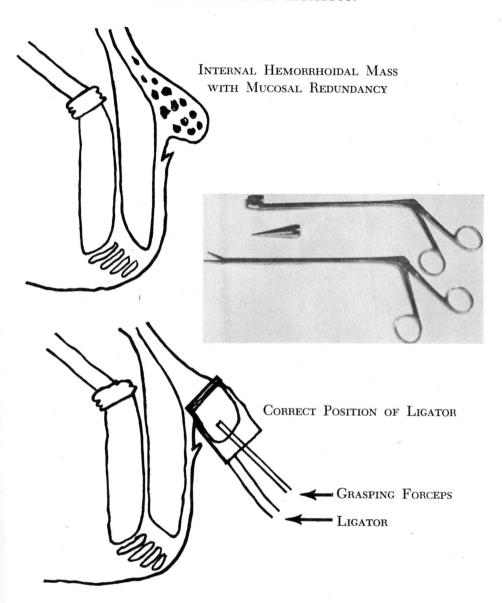

INTERNAL HEMORRHOIDAL MASS
WITH MUCOSAL REDUNDANCY

CORRECT POSITION OF LIGATOR

←— GRASPING FORCEPS

←— LIGATOR

INJECTION THERAPY

In this technique a sclerosing agent of 5% phenol in oil or quinine urea hydrochloride is injected into the hemorrhoidal mass well above the mucocutaneous line. This creates schlerosing of the vessels and fibrous tissue formation to cause the mucosa to adhere to the muscularis. I personally feel that this technique is cumbersome, nonspecific, incomplete, and has been superseded in many practices by the banding techniques.

CLAMP AND CAUTERY RADIAL TECHNIQUE

This is one of the historically oldest techniques, and one of the most frequently used by men who have become very proficient in this procedure. In the cautery technique the hemorrhoids are encompassed in a hemorrhoidal clamp and excised from the top of the clamp. The mucosal and skin edges are cauterized from the top of the clamp. A suture is placed at the apical area of the hemorrhoid, and this suture is run to and fro beneath the clamp down to the anorectal line and tied. The clamp is then removed. This is repeated on all hemorrhoids visible. Any crypts that appear suspicious are cauterized, and an internal sphincterotomy is performed by either a sharp blade or the cautery tip. The wound edges of the anoderm are then beveled as smoothly as possible and extended well beyond the anal verge for adequate drainage.

I personally prefer other techniques, for the following reasons:

1. the excessive amount of burn and damaged tissue

2. the slough of tissue in 5 to 7 days with the attendant bleeding

3. the higher incidence of stenosis

CLAMP AND SUTURE RADIAL TECHNIQUE

In this technique the patient is under general anesthesia and placed in an exaggerated lithotomy position. The perirectal area is painted with Mercresin, and sterile drapes are applied.

The anus is gently divulged with the examining finger, and then the anal region is infiltrated in four quadrants with Xylocaine 0.5% and epinephrine. The lubricated Muir operating speculum is then inserted into the rectum, noting the hemorrhoidal masses usually at the right anterior, right posterior, and left lateral positions. These three hemorrhoidal masses are then removed in sequence in the following manner:

One Allis forcep is placed on the skin tag, if present, and one is placed on the internal hemorrhoidal mass. This tissue is then elevated with the Allis forceps and the skin tag is cut free to the anorectal line with Mayo scissors. A curved Oschner clamp is placed over the internal hemorrhoidal mass while the mass is elevated from the muscularis by the traction on the Allis forceps. At this point the Allis forceps are removed from the hemorrhoidal mass. A Mayo-Hegar needle driver is used to place an #0 plain (#864 Ethicon) suture under the Oschner clamp about ¼″ from the tip of the clamp and is tied, compressing the tissue under the tip of the clamp.

This suture is not cut but is run to and fro below the clamp down to the anorectal line and then to and fro back up to the original knot. At this point, while gently pulling on the suture, the Oschner clamp is slowly removed and the suture tied, using the loose suture end of the original knot. Oozing of blood in the elliptical external wound can usually be controlled with light electrocoagulation. If a larger vessel is bleeding, it may be necessary to insert a hemostatic #0 plain suture or so.

1. Some physicians use a clamp above and below the anorectal line. I feel that using a clamp on the anoderm causes a crush type injury with resultant tissue trauma, edema, and unnecessary pain to the patient.

2. Some physicians close the eliptical anodermal wound with #000 chromic suture. I find this causing suture discomfort, edema, induration, and do not do so.

3. Inflamed crypts may be elevated with a crypt hook and snipped off.

4. In order to relieve postoperative sphincter spasm or a stenotic anus, a posterior sphincterotomy is often performed. This should not be done without experience. The mucosa is divided in the posterior midline with a #15 Bard Parker blade exposing the sphincter fibers. *A FEW* of these fibers are bisected *longitudinally* (at a right angle to the fibers).

5. Fissures if present are often excised during this procedure. See discussion on fissures.

6. Fistulae and abscesses are sometimes done in conjunction with this procedure. See discussion on fistulae and abscesses.

7. Some physicians use no clamp at all, relying on their suturing celerity alone to control bleeding.

CRYOHEMORRHOIDECTOMY

Cryosurgery destroys tissue by freezing it: These are three different modalities in common usage:

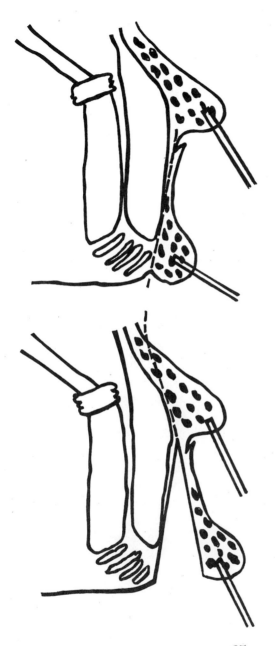

CLAMP AND SUTURE TECHNIQUE

Internal and External
Hemorrhoids with
Allis Forceps
Applying Traction

Dotted line shows
incision path of
curved Mayo
scissors to a
point above the
anorectal line.

External Mass
Excised by Mayo
Scissors

Dotted line shows
where the curved
Oschner clamp
will be placed.

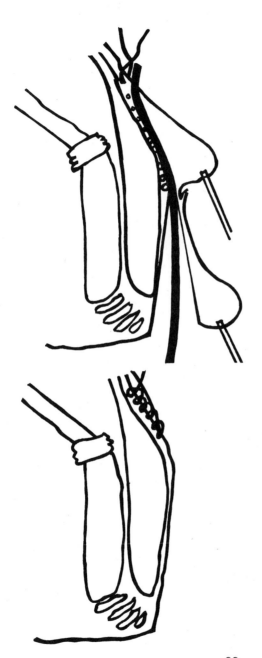

CLAMP AND SUTURE TECHNIQUE

Heavy dark line
represents curved
Oschner clamp in
position.

NOTE: Suture placed
at the tip of the
clamp. This suture
is tied and then
run to and fro
beneath the clamp
(small circles°)
to a point just
above the crypt
line. It is then
passed to and fro
beneath the clamp
back to the tip of
the clamp, at which
point the clamp is
removed as the
suture is gently
pulled. The suture
is then tied at
the original knot.

1. liquid nitrogen ($-196°C$)
2. nitrous oxide
3. carbon dioxide

In this technique the cryoprobe is held on the tissue to be destroyed for two to three minutes.

I do not like this procedure, for the following reasons:

1. It is not painless on application, especially when used on the anodermal lesions. Many men find that they must infiltrate the tissues with local anesthetic first.

2. There is much edema after this procedure, which is bothersome and difficult to explain to the patient. There is also marked discomfort associated with this edema.

3. There is copious seromucous discharge after this procedure that lasts for weeks.

I have found one fine use for the cryoprobe, however. In cases of resistant pruritus ani, when I have been unable to attain relief for the patient, I use the cryoprobe anteriorly and posteriorly on both sides of the anal verge and have found that this affords the patient marked remission of the pruritus.

MUCOSAL TUBE RESECTION
(Modified Whitehead)

This technique should be attempted only by experienced, qualified physicians and then only in cases of marked prolapse, for which it well may be, if done correctly, the procedure of choice.

In cases with a "doughnut" prolapse an elliptoid incision is made about the anal verge halfway to the edge of the prolapse-anoderm margin. Six Adair Allis forceps are placed equilaterally on the mucosal edge of this incision. The index finger is inserted into the rectum, grasping all six forceps under traction. The resultant mucosal tube with the hemorrhoidal venous plexus attached and visible is then carefully dissected from the outlying structures with Mayo scissors and gauze finger pushing.

This dissection is carried to the level of the apex of the hemorrhoids. Four straight hemostats are used at the four quadrants to mark this level. The mucosal tube is then excised below the hemostats. The hemostats are removed one by one as the Adair Allis forceps are placed on the free mucosal edge in an equilateral fashion. This free annular mucosal edge is then tacked to the ring of anoderm with 6 to 8 #0 Dexon sutures. This new anorectal line is then anastomosed with #000 chromic sutures, removing the Adair Allis forceps as the surgeon proceeds with the suturing. If done correctly, the new anorectal line should be at the level of a normal anorectal line by the next morning.

If done incorrectly, there will be an extension of mucosa in the anal verge, resulting in a wet anus due to mucoid secretion. This is known as a "whitehead defect" and must later be cauterized in order that scar tissue supplant the secreting mucosa.

In short, this technique takes up the longitudinal mucosal redundancy, while the other techniques take up radial redundancy.

DILATION

In this technique, under general anesthesia, the anus is extremely dilated to the point of squeezing an entire hand into the orifice. This creates scar tissue to adhere the mucosa to the muscularis and to sclerose the venous plexus. This is the one technique for hemorrhoids that I cannot bring myself to try. I feel that it is simply too traumatic a procedure to accomplish what is to be done.

LASER

At some future date when less expensive, less cumbersome, laser units are available, this modality may be adapted for hemorrhoidal surgery. It would have several advantages:

1. The beam seals small vessels as it cuts through them.

2. The burn area is only a cell or two layers thick.

3. There would be minimal edema.

4. There would be practically no suturing.

5. It is a very precise excision done through a microscopic lens.

I did some work with a laser unit (not on humans) several years ago, and still hold out hope for its utilization in rectal work.

EXTERNAL THROMBOTIC "HEMORRHOIDS"

6

IF THE INTERNAL hemorrhoidal plexus is large enough and dilated enough and has enough forced pressure it will rupture and an amount of blood will be forced into the anodermal area as an external clot. This is swollen, painful, and usually of a bluish hue. Its size may vary from 2-3 mm. to a circumanal "doughnut" associated with marked mucosal prolapse. In 7 to 10 days it will atrophy into a skin tag.

If this has occurred one or two days before the patient presents himself, I ask the patient how the present discomfort compares with yesterday's discomfort. If the patient feels much better and it hardly bothers him, except for the swelling, I do nothing except explain to the patient that this is a sign that his internal hemorrhoids need attention. I reexamine the patient several days later. If, however, this external clot is still causing much discomfort to the patient, the clot should be excised. This is a very simple office procedure.

The dome of the external clot is infiltrated with 0.5 cc. of Xylocaine, 1% with epinephrine. (This is injected into the epidermis until blanching occurs from the epinephrine; it is not injected deeper into the clot.) A #15 Bard Parker blade is used to incise the tissue over the clot for a length of about half the diameter of the clot. At this point the clot usually pops out. If it does not extrude it may be extracted by inserting a mosquito hemostat into it and then pulling it out. Instrumentation, however, should be kept at a minimum. Do not try to extract all smaller clots from the lobulated tissue or the patient may, due to trauma, have marked prolapse by the following day.

An alternate method, after the injection of the local anesthetic, follows: The dome of the skin over the clot is grasped with an Allis forceps, and, as this tissue is elevated, a pair of curved scissors is used to cut away the tissue below the Allis forceps. This results in a larger elliptical wound for better drainage.

In either of these methods:

1. Simple pressure for 3 minutes will stop most bleeding, and the patient is so instructed.

2. Occasionally it is necessary to touch a couple of bleeding spots with an electrocautery unit. Suture is rarely needed.

3. The patient is given a prescription for an anesthetic ointment such as Diothane.

4. The patient is advised to sit in a warm tub of water for 10 min. T.I.D. *beginning the next day* and to limit activity for a few hours.

5. It is made clear to the patient that, by removing this clot, only first aid has been given and that the internal hemorrhoidal plexus needs attention.

ANAL SKIN TAGS

Skin tags are:

1. the result of a previous external hemorrhoidal clot,

2. hypertrophied anal skin fold from chronic pruritus ani,

3. a sequelae of previous rectal surgery where the wound edges healed improperly,

4. the buildup of tissue at the outer edge of fissure even though the fissure itself may have healed.

TREATMENT

During anoplastic procedures under general anesthetic these may simply be excised.

In the office after ligation or previous hospital anoplastic procedures, if these bother the patient or are the source of pruritus they may be excised under local anesthetic.

The tissue under the skin tag is infiltrated with 1% Xylocaine with epinephrine and the skin tag is elevated with an Allis forceps and excised with curved scissors. Hemostasis may be obtained with pressure and electrofulgeration. Suture is rarely necessary. Diothane ointment (or other topical anesthetic) is prescribed for the patient. Sitz baths at home may be instituted on the following day if there is no bleeding.

73

PROCTITIS AND CRYPTITIS

CAUSES

1. Diet—the foods generally listed for pruritus ani
2. Neoplasm
3. Hemorrhoids
4. Mucosal redundancy
5. Diarrhea
6. Constipation
7. Inflammatory bowel disease
8. Radiation (factitial proctitis)

TREATMENT

1. Eradication of hemorrhoids and/or mucosal redundancy.
2. Anusal H.C. suppositories B.I.D. (Personally, I prefer a similar suppository with benzocaine.)
3. Proctofoam H.C. B.I.D.
4. Correction of underlying systemic pathology.

ANAL FISSURE

An anal fissure is the result of:

1. proctitis
2. anal stenosis
3. large stool
4. trauma

It is a tear of the mucocutaneous portions of the anal areas. As it persists the pulsion force of stool passage results in a buildup of tissue at its external, wedge-shaped pole. This bulging tissue build-up is called a sentinel node of Brodie.

An anal fissure is associated with painful bowel movements with bleeding at stool.

If there is no sentinel node, that is, if the fissure is early in development, it will often heal after dilation of the anal verge and cauterization of the fissure itself with 50% trichloroacetic acid. No local anesthetic is needed for this, although the patient will experience some transitory discomfort. If there is a sentinel node present it usually must be removed to accomplish healing.

The skin tag and fissure areas are infiltrated with 1% Xylocaine. The tag is then grasped with an Allis forceps and the skin tag excised with curved scissors. The indurated lateral edges are also trimmed off, and the fissure itself then lightly cauterized with 50% trichloroacetic acid or an electrocoagulation unit.

Needless to say, the underlying cause for the fissure must be eliminated by either or several of the following to prevent recurrence:

stool softeners

Anusol H.C. suppositories for the proctitis

sphincterotomy for stenosis

eradication of hemorrhoidal disease

cessation of anal sex habits

It is best to place the patient on an anesthetic ointment after treating a fissure.

ANAL FISSURE WITH A SENTINEL NODE
AT THE OUTER MARGIN

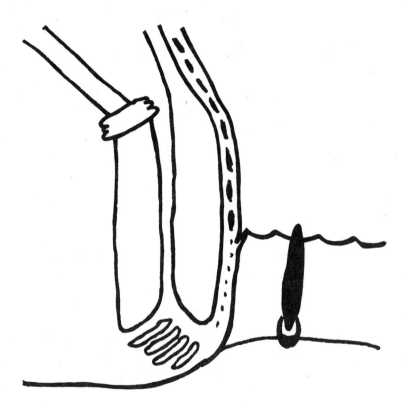

HYPERTROPHIED ANAL PAPILLAE

These are inflammatory polypoid lesions arising from the anal crypts. They are caused by proctitis and cryptitis of long duration. Hypertrophied papillae vary in size. I have seen them as large as my thumb.

TREATMENT

Smaller papillae sometimes decrease in size after the proctitis is effectively treated. Usually, however, they must be fulgerated or excised. At the surgical table, under general anesthesia, it is a simple matter to excise or fulgerate them. In the office situation they may be removed with scissors under local anesthetic. In this situation an electrocautery unit should be in readiness because bleeding is occasionally brisk.

FISTULAE AND ABSCESSES

Proctitis usually extends into the anorectal crypts, resulting in a cryptitis. This inflammation advances into the crypt glands and then in some cases will dissect as a tract through the soft tissues to form an abscess in an area nearby. This tract is called a fistula.

Fistulae are classed by their external opening on the skin surface in relation to the anus.

| Anterior | Type I | |
| Anterolateral | Type II | Right or Left |

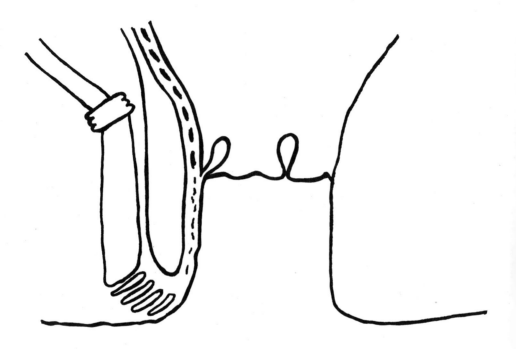

External Thrombotic "Hemorrhoids"

Midline Laterally	Type III	Right or Left
Posterolateral	Type IV	Right or Left
Posterior	Type V	Right or Left

Note that these are not termed one o'clock, twelve o'clock, etc., as this varies with the positioning of the patient.

There are four classifications of abscesses depending on their location to the rectum:

1. subcutaneous   (in perirectal space)
2. ischiorectal   (in ischiorectal space)
3. supralevator   (in supralevator space)
4. submural   (between the mucosa and muscularis cephalad from the crypt line)

Because fistulae do not dissect through fascia if soft tissue is an alternative, I feel that supralevator abscess formation occurs through extension up the space of the posterior anal triangle, which is a potential space due to the gap in the rectococcygeus and pubococcygeus musculature (Brick's space). It is due to this philosophy that I believe supralevator abscesses should be drained by an incision posterior to the anal ring musculature in this posterior anal triangle rather than laterally over the ischiorectal space. An incision here merely creates a secondary fistula through the levator ani.

POINTS IN FISTULA AND ABSCESS SURGERY

1. The mandatory immediate treatment of an acute anorectal abscess is incision and drainage. This is an office procedure.

CLASSIFICATION OF ABSCESSES

ANTERIOR

I

II   II

ISCHIAL   III   III   ISCHIAL
TUBEROSITY   TUBEROSITY

IV   IV

V

POSTERIOR

Local anesthetic is infiltrated into the skin over a fluctuant area of the abscess, and a #15 Bard Parker blade is used to make a 1 cm. incision into the abscess cavity. A mosquito hemostat may be spread inside this cavity to facilitate drainage. The purulent drainage is captured on gauze or cellucotton sponges. The gloved hand of the surgeon is used to grasp these sponges as the glove is removed incorporating the sponges inside the removed glove. A knot is then tied in the wrist end of the glove. This keeps the office free of most of the offensive odor of the saturated sponges.

2. After the incision and drainage the patient is placed on Keflex 250 mg. Q.I.D. (if no allergy is present) and sitz baths. The patient should then be scheduled for definitive surgery in 7 to 10 days (after the acute inflammation has subsided).

3. Definitive surgery should be left to experienced, capable hands.

4. At surgery a large cruciate incision is made over the abscess cavity and the four resultant right-angle skin tabs are excised. All of the necrotic tissue in the abscess cavity (appearing as grayish-yellow adipose tissue) must be debrided by sharp and blunt dissection. In most instances a probe may be passed through the fistulous tract to the crypt line. If the fistula does not pass through sphincter musculature (that is, a superficial subcutaneous fistula), the overlying tissue is marsupalized to the probe and debrided of necrotic tissue. If the fistulous tract lies at a level where it is deeper than sphincter musculature I no longer feel that the sphincter musculature should be bisected. Rather, a stretched-out gauze sponge is passed through the fistulous tract into the rectal vault. This rough sponge is used to scarify the necrotic lining of the fistulous tract with a sawing motion. The sponge is then removed. The internal opening at

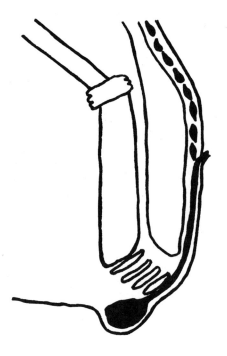

SUBCUTANEOUS

SUBMURAL

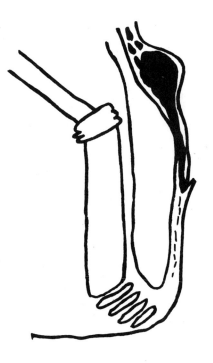

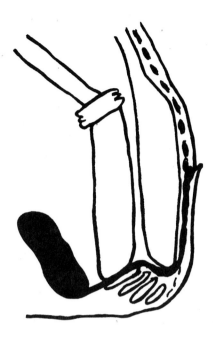

ISCHIORECTAL

SUPRALEVATOR

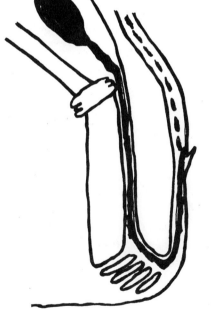

the crypt line is closed with #000 chromic suture. Then, from the outside, the fistulous tract and abscess cavity are packed with continuous ¼″ iodoform gauze, which is to be removed the next morning. Occasionally, an internal opening of a fistulous tract cannot be found or demonstrated. In this instance, I no longer feel that an artificial one should capriciously be made. This only creates a fistulous tract to satisfy the surgeon.

5. The postoperative care of an abscess cavity is extremely important and must be constantly monitored by the surgeon. Postoperative care on my service includes:

> sitz baths
>
> Keflex 250mg. Q.I.D. P.O. (unless allergic)
>
> irrigation of abscess cavity with saline and/or H_2O
>
> chloromycetin-elase ointment instilled into the cavity twice daily

PROCIDENTIA

This is a result of an incontinence of the supportive musculature of the rectal vault. It is usually found in very young children and/or elderly patients. Procidentia is a prolapse of the rectal muscularis and mucosa, while rectal prolapse is merely a prolapse of the rectal mucosa. It may be differentiated not only by the greater prolapsed mass, but also by the fact that in prolapse there are radial creases in the annular mass, while in procidentia annular folds are presented.

DIVERTICULAR DISEASE 7

DIVERTICULI are discovered in about 10% of routine barium enemas. This incidence increases to about 40% in advancing age. They are most often in the sigmoid colon and less often present progressing cephalad in the colon. Diverticuli are outpouchings of the colonic mucosa through weak areas in the circular muscle caused by increased intraluminal pressure. Irritable colon syndrome may be an etiological factor in the development of this condition. Radiography reveals long narrow conical deformity with a normal mucosal pattern thrown up in folds.

Symptoms occur in about 10% of diverticular patients. Occasionally, a diverticulum will get a fecal bolus in it, causing a peridiverticulitis. This inflammation may proceed to fistulous formation to contiguous organs (dysuria in a diverticulitis patient may indicate urinary-colonic fistulization), or even to perforation, with peritonitis and abscess formation. Inflammatory luminal obstruction may also occur.

Diverticular disease should be surgically treated once an intractable stage has been reached, in an effort to prevent these dire complications.

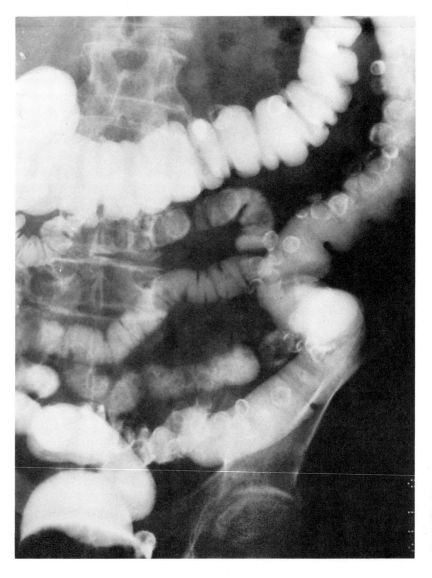

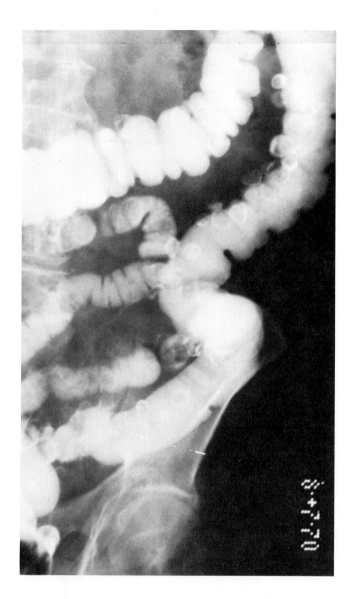

DIVERTICULOSIS

NOTE: Characteristic outpouching and spasm.

ULCERATIVE COLITIS 8

Definition

ULCERATIVE COLITIS is an acute, subacute, or chronic, idiopathic, progressive, occasionally fulminating, inflammatory disease of the large bowel characterized by periods of exacerbation and quiescence.

Incidence

It occurs equally in both sexes and in all races. It usually begins in the teens, twenties, or thirties, but has been found to be present in six-week- and four-month-old infants. The human appears to be the only creature suffering from this disease. Occasionally, a family may show a susceptibility to ulcerative colitis.

TYPES

There are several classifications:

A. (Dr. Bockus)

1. *Relapsing Remitting Type*
   a. mild to severe
   b. rectum and rectosigmoid involved
   c. lasts 4-12 weeks
   d. usually self-limiting

2. *Chronic Continous Type*
   a. rectum and entire colon involved
   b. 6 months and longer
   c. fibrotic deterioration

3. *Acute Fulminating Type*
   a. descending or entire colon involved
   b. poor nutrition, bleeding, ulceration, dilation of colon
   c. hyperpyrexia

B. (Dr. Cantor)

1. *Acute Fulminating Ulcerative Colitis*:
   a. mild, diffuse inflammation of the mucous membrane
   b. smooth, friable, reddened mucosal surface that bleeds with the slightest trama

2. *Acute Recurring Ulcerative Colitis*

   Numerous miliary (pinhead) abscesses appear as tiny yellow spots seen through an edematous, reddened mucosal surface. The abscesses lie in the deeper layers of the mucous membrane.

3. *Chronic Ulcerative Colitis*

   Mucosa is diffusely reddened and granular (it appears moth-eaten). Petecchial hemorrhages are present and the mucosa bleeds readily. This stage is associated with diarrhea

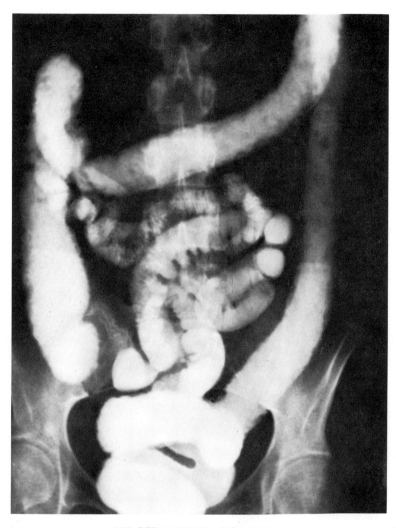

ULCERATIVE COLITIS
NOTE: Cobblestone appearance
              Mucosal ulcerations
              Pseudopolyps
              Shortening
              Loss of haustrations

containing mucous, blood, and pus. There may be in this stage a massive loss of mucosal lining.

4. *Mild Ulcerative Colitis* (Remission Stage)

Mucosa is granular and glazed. There is little or no bleeding; the mucosa is no longer hemorrhagic. There is a mucopurulent debris adherent to the bowel wall.

ETIOLOGY

Causes of Recurrence

Many causes have been expanded but none proven as single causes. Most are considered etiological factors.

1. bacterial origin

2. viral

3. familial (In some families there seems to be an inherent susceptibility to ulcerative colitis.)

4. primary biological factor lack

5. allergy, especially eggs, chocolate, wheat, and milk "allergy" (probably lactose deficit, which complicates ulcerative colitis)

6. autoimmunity (Mucosa damaged by various agents—bacteria and/or viral—and mucosal particles became antigenic and elicit systemic antibodies, which react with material similar to the antigen and cause more damage.)

7. psychological factors—possibly as much a cause as any, with one or all of the following:

a.   shyness and withdrawal
b.   rigidity, obsessions, perfectionism
c.   feeling of insecurity and diffuse anxiety
d.   feeling of frustration—not able to live up to unrealistic self-images
e.   poor sex adjustment
f.   feeling of helplessness or hopelessness

The following factors have caused a recurrence of ulcerative colitis:

infection elsewhere
other surgery
antibiotics
pregnancy
menstruation
dietary indiscretions
fatigue (physical and mental)
leaving home
sexual conflicts
economic problems
fear (or loss) of an important person in one's life

SYMPTOMS

Early—loose stools with fatigue

Late—frequent bloody, loose, mucoid stools with pus. Abdominal pain not as frequent as mild cramps and discomfort. Other symptoms are anorexia, weakness, nausea, amenorrhea in females, cramps and pain in lower left quadrant.

PATHOLOGY

Progresses from the rectum (crypts are the fundamental lesion site) retroperistaltically in 95% of cases. The mucosa is inflamed and friable, with scattered small bleeding points and minute ulcers. These ulcers become confluent and the colon may become denuded of mucosa and perforation may occur. Pseudopolypsis may also occur in later stages.

Associated Systemic Findings and Complications

Anemia

Amenorrhea in females

Stomatitis

Thrombophlebitis

Arthritis

Amyloidosis

Loss of potassium

Loss of protein

Iriditis

Uveitis

Iridocyclitis

Clubbed fingers

Hepatitis

Myocardial damage

Fissure

Fistulae

Fistulization with other organs results in:

1. fecal breath and vomiting

2. reversal of A/G ratio

3. sudden increase in diarrhea

Toxic megacolon (usually from overzealous use of anticholinergics) results in an increase in temperature and sudden constipation, with abdominal distension caused by involvement of main muscular coats, with loss of muscles and destruction of Auerbach's plexus and ganglion cells.

Perforation—May be "silent."

One survey found 6% of ulcerative colitis with simultaneous ankylosing spondylitis but made no interpretation.

Stricture, pseudopolyposis, and malignancy are more frequent as the involved segment progresses from the rectum to the cecum.

DIAGNOSIS

1. 90-95% diagnosed by proctosigmoidoscopy

2. history of mucosanguinous diarrhea

3. radiographic findings:

  a. very early—nothing

  b. then signs of spasms and irritability

  c. later loss of haustrations resulting in a "lead pipe" appearance (A barium enema is considered contradicted if there is evidence of mucosal slough or severe ulceration.)

DIFFERENTIAL DIAGNOSIS

Bacteria:
    Shigella
    Salmonella   stool analysis and culture

Parasites:
    Endamœba Histolytica

Polyarteritis, other collagen disease: biopsy

Malignancy: biopsy, barium enema, colonoscopy, sigmoidoscopy

Granulomatous Colitis (Crohn's disease)

	ULCERATIVE COLITIS	GRANULOMATOUS COLITIS
Usual Location	Left Colon	Right Colon
Small Bowel Involvement	Rare	Common
Rectal Involvement	Over 90%	Under 20%
Transanal Bleeding	Common	Rare
Stricture	Rare	Common
Perforation	Occasional	Rare
Fistulous Formation	Unusual	Common
Pseudopolyps	Common	Never
Malabsorption Syndrome	Never	Common

INCIDENCE OF ASSOCIATED MALIGNANCY

Normal population has cancer of colon in 0.1%.

One study:

Years of ulcerative colitis	% Cancer
0-9	0.4
10-19	2.0
20-29	5.8

Another study:

Years of Ulcerative Colitis	% Cancer
Under 10	3.8
Over 10	45.5

Another study:

Years of Ulcerative Colitis	% Cancer
0	0.1
8	1.6
15	4.5
20	12.6

Proctology

In Summary

1. There is a greater incidence of cancer in patients with ulcerative colitis.

2. The longer and/or more severe the ulcerative colitis, the greater the incidence of cancer.

3. There is a greater incidence of cancer in ulcerative colitis patients with pseudopolyps, even though these are seldom malignant themselves.

4. Ulcerative colitis is considered a premalignant disease.

5. Colectomy should be performed in all patients with ulcerative colitis with pseudopolyposes and with intractibility.

Treatment

1. DIET: Some cases must have nothing by mouth while others may have a bland, low-residue, high-protein, high-calorie diet.

These patients should have *NO*:

> Highly seasoned foods
> Liquor
> Carbonated beverages
> Orange juice (grape juice OK)
> Seeds
> Condiments
> Cucumbers
> Milk
> Chocolate

Wheat
Eggs
Raw fruit
Raw vegetables
Spices
Radishes
Onions

2. Absolute bed rest unless the patients have a very mild case.

3. Sedation.

4. Tranquilizers.

5. Vitamins—especially B complex, C for tissue repair, and K.

6. Anabolic drugs.

7. Fluids as necessary.

8. Protein hydrolysates.

9. Iron and/or blood as necessary.

10. Sitz baths.

11. Psyllium seeds.

12. Broad spectrum antibiotics may cause diarrhea; use only if deep ulcers are present or an increase in temperature occurs; then use parenterally only.

13. Azulfidine appears to be the best drug in ulcerative colitis. Three to four 0.5gm. tablets Q.I.D. Follow each dose with 12 ozs. water. Taper off slowly. Sulfa drugs in ulcerative colitis have unmasked a systemic lupus erythematosis in several cases.

14. Neomycin may be used if the patient is sensitive to Azulfidine.

15. Anticholinergics should be used very cautiously due to possible colonic distension and development of toxic megacolon.

16. Psychiatric therapy is considered questionable by many authors, especially in adults, but at the same time it is bound to help at least many of the underlying psychic disturbances.

17. Opiates should be used only for short periods if necessary, due to the possibility of masking a perforation.

18. Steriods: Better than ACTH since ACTH depends on the patient's own adrenal reserves. Steriods should be used IV or IM rather than orally, but a close check must be kept on serum potassium and calcium. Medrol enpacks and cortenemas are superb. Steriods are contraindicated in perforation, peritonitis, severe anemia, electrolytic inbalance.

19. Surgery (abdominal—perineal).

CANCER OF THE COLON AND RECTUM 19

THIS YEAR about a hundred thousand people will be found to have carcinoma of the colon and rectum. This represents the largest incidence of cancer of the human race except skin cancer. More than half of these patients will die as the result of this disease. Only lung cancer causes more deaths in the malignant field. This is truly tragic, because only 10% of the cases should expire from this disease. These sorry statistics are primarily due to the lack of early diagnosis, resulting from the assumption of the patient (and often the physician) that the symptoms and signs of cancer of the large bowel and rectum are merely due to hemorrhoids, which unfortunately present the same symptoms or signs. The essential diagnostic methods for the early discovery of cancer of the rectum and colon are:

1. Visual examination

2. Palpation

3. Proctosigmoidoscopy

4. Barium enema

5. Colonoscopy

Almost half of the patients with cancer of the large bowel have distant metastases or extensive local spread, when first seen. It is disturbing to find that so many patients complaining of bleeding from the rectum, severe constipation, and cramps in the lower abdomen have been treated symptomatically without the benefit of a physical examination. Seventy-one percent of the malignancies of the colon and rectum are within reach of the sigmoidoscope.

0-8 cm.	13%
9-15 cm.	43%
16-20 cm.	10%
21-25 cm.	5%
Over 25 cm.	29%

The prognosis in carcinoma of the colon and rectum is brighter for adults than for children, and more favorable as the sight of the cancer moves cephalad from the anal canal. Prognosis should take into consideration the extent of tumor spread, as noted in Duke's classification and survival rate. This is a five-year survival rate.

Type A: The lesion is limited to the mucosa. 100%

Type B₁: The lesion extends into the muscularis but does not penetrate it, and the regional nodes are negative. 66.6%

Type B₂: The lesion penetrates through the muscularis with negative nodes. 53.9%

Type C₁: The lesion is limited to the wall with positive
nodes.   42.8%

Type C₂: The lesion is through all layers with positive nodes. 22.4%

Periodic digital, proctosigmoidoscopic, barium enema, and colonoscopic examination are a necessity after surgery for cancer of the colon and rectum to detect recurrent or new lesions.

SYMPTOMS AND SIGNS OF CARCINOMA

Many carcinomas will exhibit no symptoms at first and will be discovered early only as part of a routine examination of the colon and rectum.

The symptoms are:

1. ill-defined abdominal discomfort or pain that tends to persist

2. the presence of blood in or on the stool (anemia indicates ulceration), which indicates that the tumor is large enough to have been growing for months

3. a palpable mass in the abdomen

4. a change from normal bowel habits to:
    a. diarrhea
    b. increasing constipation and diarrhea
    c. alternating constipation and diarrhea
    d. decreased caliber of stool
    e. sensation of incomplete evacuation
    f. increasing flatus

5. unexplained loss of weight
6. unexplained anemia

Severe symptoms such as great weight loss, cachexia, jaundice, hepar enlargement, extreme malnutrition and dehydration are signs of advanced carcinoma.

SYMPTOMS OF RIGHT COLON CARCINOMA

1. pain
2. anemia—pallor, fatigue, weakness, dizziness, dyspnea (severe anemia from right colon cancer is less serious in prognosis than from left colon cancer)
3. tumor mass—first sign in 10%—cancer until proven otherwise

SYMPTOMS OF LEFT COLON CARCINOMA

1. obstruction
2. bleeding
3. change in bowel habits
4. decrease in stool caliber

SYMPTOMS OF RECTAL CARCINOMA

1. bleeding—most common sign
2. a sensation of incomplete evacuation
3. tenesmus (indicates involvement of sphincter)
4. mucous diarrhea
5. pain (late)

BENIGN POLYPS OF THE COLON AND RECTUM

ADENOMA

This is the most common type of polyp, representing 85% of all the polyps in the rectum and colon. They may be single or multiple, sessile or pedunculated, or minute to obstructive in size. The lesions are multiple in 25% to 30% of the patients. Malignant transformation occurs in 15% of these polyps. The most common symptoms with simple adenosis is bleeding. It should be noted that 20% to 40% of of polyps are missed by barium enema and sigmoidoscopic examination.

VILLOUS POLYPS

These are the second most common type of polyp found in 15% of the total study of polyps and are mostly in the rectum and low sigmoid. These are spongy in consistency, and secrete large amounts of mucus. They are rarely pedunculated. Malignancy in these may be indicated by ulceration of the lesion. Villous polyps tend to recur after removal. They have a high malignant potential (30%). Diagnosis of malignant change can be made only after excision and study of the *entire* tumor specimen.

MALIGNANT LESIONS OF THE COLON AND RECTUM

ADENOCARCINOMA

This is the most common malignant lesion, and undergoes lymphatic spread earlier in the left colon. The lesions are bulky with rolled margins that form a sharp demarcation. Circumferential

105

ADENOCARCINOMA

NOTE: Concentric constriction resulting in an "apple core" deformity; "shelfing."

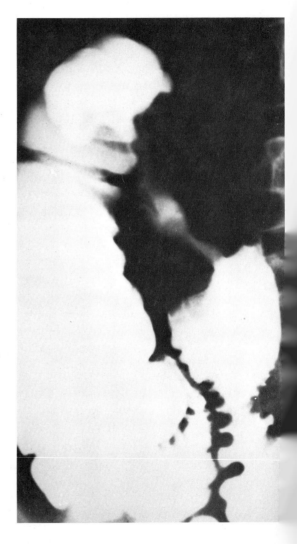

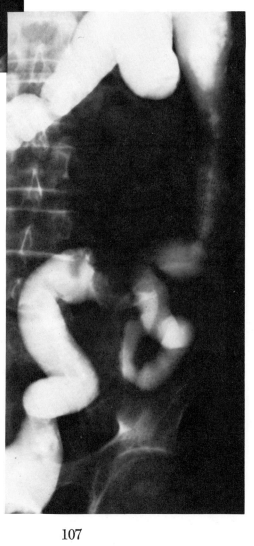

growth is more common in the left than in the right colon. Left colon lesions invade the bowel wall rapidly, while right colon lesions grow into the lumen.

LINITIS PLASTICA VARIANT

This is a very rare, and very malignant lesion infiltrating upward and downward in the bowel wall. The walls of the bowel become rigid, thick, and hard. A surface lesion is rare, although the mucosa is pebbled in appearance.

CARCINOID TUMORS

These are usually found in the appendix, ileocecal region, distal ileal segment, rectum, and cecum. Often multiple; slow in growing, with a yellowish tinge.

SARCOMATOUS TUMORS

These are rare but highly malignant. The local growth is slow but rapidly invades blood vessels. Metastasis is usually by the venous system. Prognosis in sarcomatous tumors is extremely poor despite treatment, due to the marked early venous metastases.

Success in treating cancer of the colon and rectum depends on early diagnosis followed by early and effective treatment. Even if sigmoidoscopy reveals no polyps, patients with a family history of polyps or those whose symptoms persist should have barium enema studies and colonoscopy. If a polyp is discovered on X ray in the colon and surgery seems indicated, the operation should not be performed until the presence of the polyp is verified by a second X ray or colonoscopy to rule out the possibility of a fecalith.

CONGENITAL MULTIPLE POLYPOSIS

This is a disease of young individuals, and unfortunately a total colectomy must be done at an early date, because carcinoma will inevitably supervene. The rectal vault may be saved if it contains no polyps and the entire remains can be viewed through a sigmoidoscope, and if the surgeon feels the patient will adhere to regular sigmoidoscopic examination for the rest of his life.

ACUTE INTESTINAL OBSTRUCTION RESULTING FROM CARCINOMA

In this patient, relief of obstruction must take place first; then detailed diagnostic studies can be carried out. It is the competence of the ileocecal valve that makes large bowel obstruction a closed-loop type of obstruction created by an obstructive lesion at one end and a competent ileocecal valve at the other. Because gas and fluid ejected into the colon from the large bowel cannot be forced back through the illeocecal valve, tremendous distention, nausea, and vomiting may result.

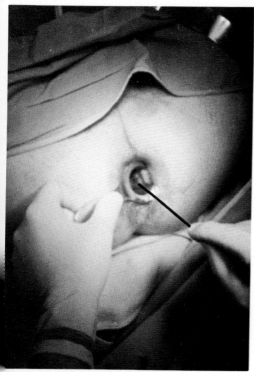

ANODERM, CRYPT LINE, AND RECTAL MUCOSA

The probe is on the tip of the crypts. Note the distinctive mucoid redness of the mucosa.

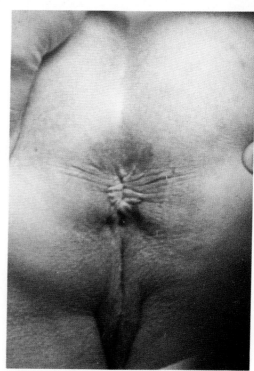

PRURITUS ANI

Note the hypertrophic anal skin folds and excoriation.

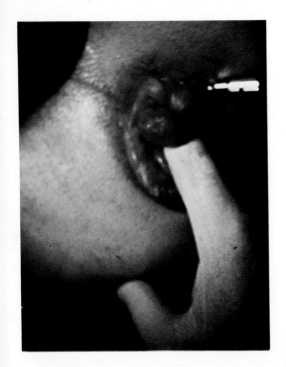

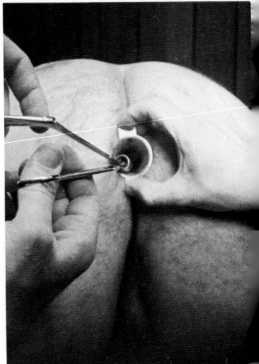

HEMORRHOIDAL LIGATION

Internal hemorrhoidal mass being pulled into cylinder prior to ligation.

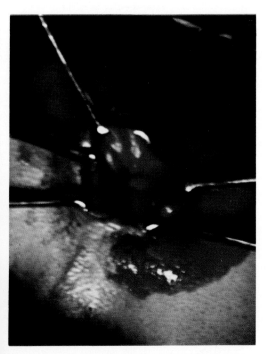

MUCOSAL TUBE RESECTION

Adair Allis in position on the circular cut mucosal edge after extirpation of the mucosal tube immediately prior to the anastomosis of mucosa and anoderm creating a new anorectal line.

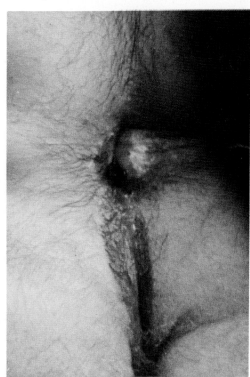

EXTERNAL THROMBOTIC "HEMORRHOID"

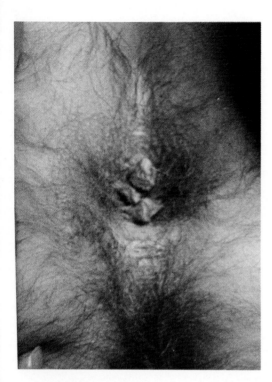

ANAL SKIN
TAGS

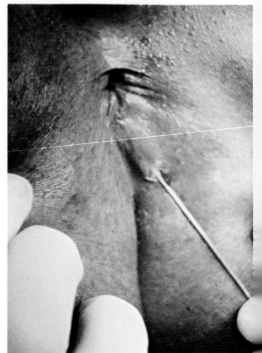

TYPE IV LEFT
ANORECTAL FISTULA

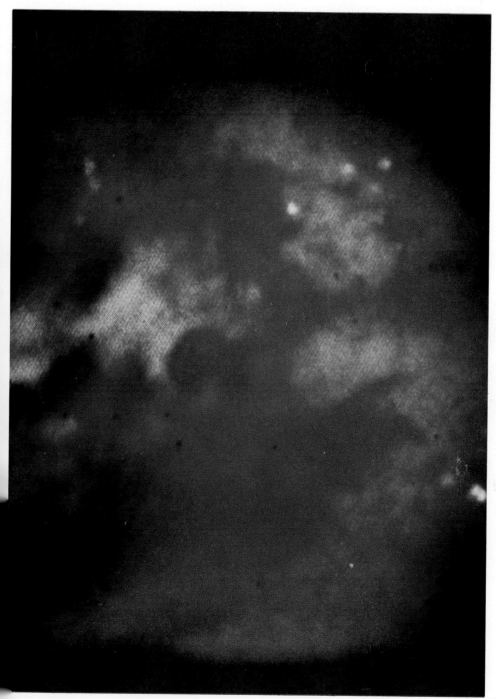

ACUTE FULMINATING ULCERATIVE COLITIS

1

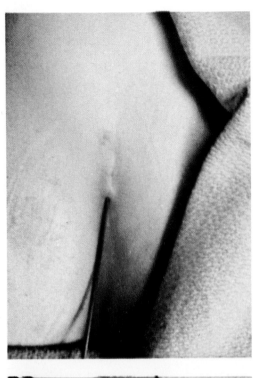

2

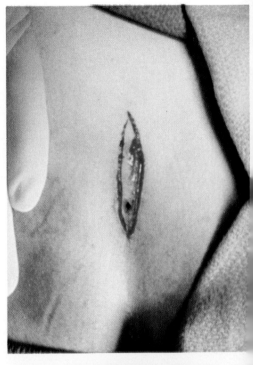

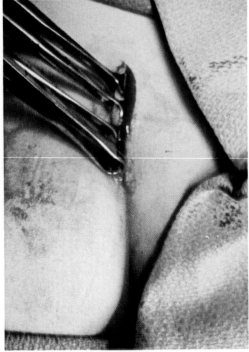

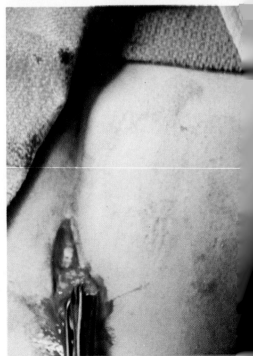

3

4

5

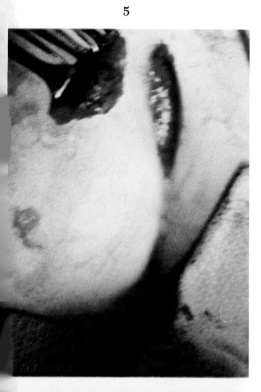

6

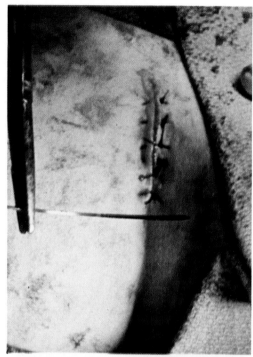

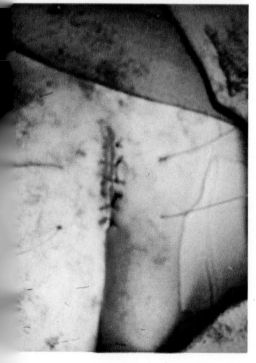

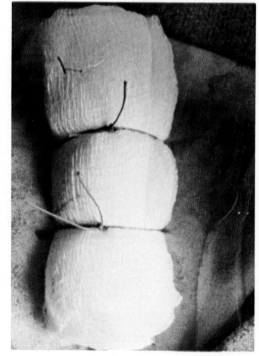

7

8

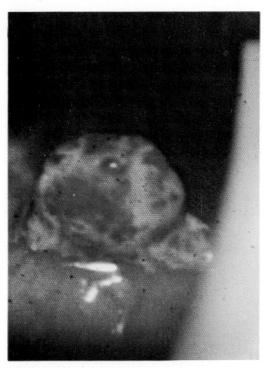

ADENOCARCINOMA

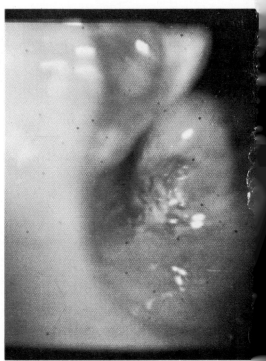

OTHER CONDITIONS 10

CONDYLOMATA ACCUMINATA

This cauliflowerlike growth is often found in the anal area and is associated with pain, discharge, and bleeding. Size may vary from a 1mm. wart to an extension over the entire perineum.

It is assumed to be a viral lesion and to be sexually transmitted. This well may be, but I feel that this does not necessarily indicate anal sex. It may be from sexually connected secretions draining to the anal region during heterosexual intercourse.

This lesion must be differentiated from:

condylomata latum—a plaquelike syphilitic lesion
carcinoma of the anus

I treat condylomata accuminata as follows:
If the lesions are not too large, I touch the tip of them with

first 50% trichloroacetic acid and then immediately with 20% Podophyllin in benzoin compound, being very careful not to get the solutions on the surrounding tissues. If this treatment is going to be effective, you will see a marked improvement in a week's time. If no improvement is noted, then, under local infiltration with 1% Xylocaine or a general anesthetic (in more massive lesions), they should be excised by the electrosurgical loop or with scissors and electrocauterization of the bases.

It should be noted that in the last few years I have had eight to ten cases of Bowen's Disease (intraepithelial carcinoma) associated with the lesions of condylomata accuminata. I believe that this was found in lesions when they extended into the mucosa of the rectum, but have not been able to prove this. At any rate I feel that tissue study should not be forgotten with condylomata accuminata and certainly utilized in persistent lesions.

HIRSCHSPRUNG'S DISEASE
(Organic Megacolon)

HISTORY

First described by Harold Hirschsprung in 1886.

DEFINITION

A dysfunction of the alimentary tract caused by a congenital total or partial aplasia of the ganglion cells of the internal nerve plexi in a larger or lesser portion of the alimentary tract.

Other Conditions

INCIDENCE

Males 3-5: 1.

HEREDITY

Appears to be an important factor, but no definite proof exists.

PATHOLOGICAL ANATOMY

Considerable dilation and hypertrophy of a larger or smaller portion of the colon (most often in sigmoid).

The rectum is usually *NOT* included in the dilation.

The ganglion cell aplasia is localized to the distal, nondilated portion of the bowel, while the dilated portion of the bowel is normal, inasmuch as the ganglion cells aplasia, as a rule, reaches up only a few centimeters into the dilated portion. The aganglionic portion is limited distally by the anus, while the proximal limit varies. (90% is in rectum or sigmoid, although it can involve the entire colon, ileum, and jejunum.)

In a few cases there is no distal narrow segment.

PATHOPHYSIOLOGY

Abnormal contractions occur in the aganglionic portion of the bowel, instead of the normal propulsive peristalsis; a constant spastic contraction of this segment occurs, which acts as an obstruction and causes dilation and hypertrophy of the proximal segment of the bowel.

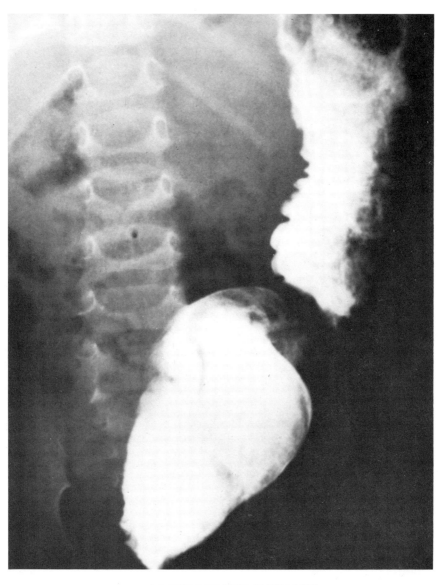

HIRSCHSPRUNG'S DISEASE
NOTE: Two short areas of involvement (sigmoid and rectum).

SYMPTOMS

NEONATAL:

1. Delayed meconium passage
2. Distension of abdomen
3. Refusal to eat
4. Vomiting
5. Intermittent intestinal obstruction

CLASSICAL (Older Children):

1. Very severe constipation
2. Distended abdomen

The severity of symptoms is proportional to the length of the aganglionic segment. The most severe symptoms are present in patients with the longest aganglionic segment.

COMPLICATIONS

Enterocolitis
Perforation
Retarded growth and development
Anemia
Water intoxication

DIAGNOSIS

History (The most important question to ask is: "Has this child ever had normal stools?")
Physical exam

115

Characteristic to have an empty rectal ampulla

X ray—variation of caliber between a distal narrow bowel portion with proximal from this, a dilated portion

Biopsy

TREATMENT

Colonic washings with N.S.

Colostomy

Drug therapy not satisfactory

Surgical removal of the aganglionic portion of the bowel

IMPACTION

An impaction is a mass of soft or hard stool in the rectal vault that has become too large for the patient to pass. It may be associated with a false diarrhea as liquid stool escapes around it.

This is usually found in three situations:

1. pediatric

2. posthemorrhoidectomy

3. geriatric

A pediatric impaction is usually due to poor bowel habits (neglecting the urge to defecate) or an anal fissure causing so much pain that the child prefers to hold back the stool. Occasionally, these tykes are presented as having "diarrhea" as the bolus causes the sphincter to be opened slightly. This "diarrhea," however, occurs with almost any movement and results in constant soilage of the skivies.

A child four to seven years old will be brought in by a nervous mother with what I have come to term a "broken home impaction." This is usually of long standing. The impaction is digitally broken up, and the mother is instructed to adminster a Fleet's enema at home. Modane liquid is given the child at bedtime nightly in slightly larger dosages than usual. This child's rectal vault has been used to the dilation caused by the impaction and therefore the sensory fibers for defecation are temporarily malfunctioning.

If the child does not have a bowel movement with the laxative given, an enema must be administered. This is repeated until the rectal vault resumes its normal function, and then the child is weaned off the laxative by gradually decreasing the dose over a period of two to three weeks. An abrupt cessation of the laxative will usually result in constipation and probably another impaction.

On rare occasions a child has not responded to the above-discussed home treatment. Admission to the pediatric hospital wing, and adherence to the same therapy for only three to four days, has resulted in normal stools. Radiographic studies in these patients often will resemble Hirschsprung's Disease.

The posthemorrhoidectomy patient, of course, has attempted to delay his first or later bowel movement in order to escape the pain that his "friends" have told him to expect. This must be prevented by the surgeon. On the first postoperative night (not surgical night) I give the patient two Dialose Plus capsules. If they have no movement the next day I discontinue the Dialose Plus and give them one Dulcolax tablet. If they have no bowel movement by noon on the third postoperative day, salt-and-soda enema is given to them with gentleness.

On dismissal from the hospital they are instructed to have a good, well-formed bowel movement each morning after taking an adjusted dose of Agarol in the evening. They are also told to take a tap water or Fleet's enema if they go two days without a bowel movement. If an impaction does occur shortly after surgery the patient will often be taken back to surgery and the impaction digitally removed under anesthesia.

The geriatric impaction case is usually due to inactivity, atonic bowel, redundant rectal mucosa, poor eating habits, and, unfortunately, occasionally the physician. Stool softeners without peristaltic agents should probably not be used in geriatric patients, as this often causes a nice, large impaction—but soft!

These people usually tolerate the digital breakup of an impaction quite well. This is followed with an enema (sometimes oil-retention) one or two Dulcolax tablets and digital reexamination the following day to confirm evacuation. The impaction-prone geriatric case usually responds to a bulk laxative like Metamucil, combined sometimes with a stool softened-peristaltic agent (Dialose Plus, etc.). Organic pathology must, of course, be ruled out as a causative factor.

FOREIGN BODIES

Patients occasionally will place almost anything into the rectal vault, usually in the quest for erotic pleasure.

Some of the items I have extracted over the years have been:

Batteries of diverse sizes
Vibrators of many sizes and parts of vibrators (one such device was still vibrating)
Small bottles

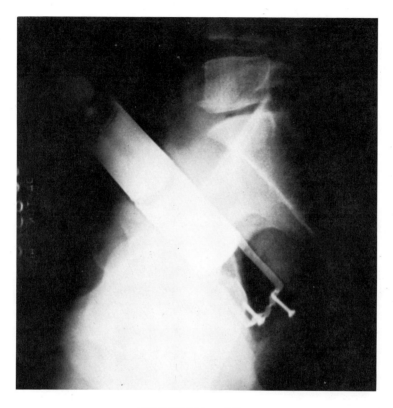

FOREIGN BODY
Res Ipsa Loquitur.

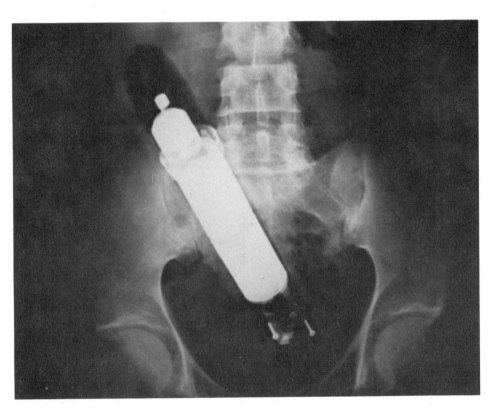

FOREIGN BODY
Res Ipsa Loquitur.

Deodorant stick cylinder
A 10 × 40 cm. hardwood painted gourd
Pencils
Assorted fruits
Enema tips

There is no standard way to extricate these items. Some may be slid out by the examining finger and some require a general anesthetic. I had to use a Lahey thyroid tenaculum to remove the gourd.

One Caution:
Some men have found light bulbs in the rectal vault. Due to the fear of breakage it is probably better to remove this by colotomy.

PROCTALGIA FUGAX

Proctalgia fugax is an intractable pain in the rectum. Many physicians feel that this is due to a painful spasm of the puborectalis muscle. This is quite rare and many other diagnoses must be ruled out before arriving at this one. Treatment consists of warm sitz baths and the digital massaging of the puborectalis muscle.

MELANOSIS COLI

This is a nonpathological observation that consists of a darkening pigmentation of the bowel wall. It is presumed to be a result of a phagocytosis of anthracene-type laxatives (i.e., cascara) in certain individuals. It is usually seen in older patients with a rather long history of constipation and laxation.

PILONIDAL CYST DISEASE

A pilonidal cyst is a cavity under the skin in the midline at the level of the buttocks. This cavity is usually filled with hair and has one or more small openings to the skin. These cysts are often not noticed until they become infected. When this occurs they become larger, painful, and full of pus. These cysts occur in about 5% of the population, in both sexes (however, about 75% of them are in males) between the ages of 15 and 25.

There is some disagreement as to the cause of these cysts and it is possible that there are really two methods of development. One is that these are congenital; that is, we are born with them. The other is that they are acquired later in life. At any rate there are several predisposing causes, such as excessive hair growth, overactive oil glands, and deep clefts between the buttocks. Trauma certainly is a factor in precipitating symptoms or activating a quiet pilonidal cyst.

Once inflammation occurs the patient will have recurring attacks, with increasing frequency and severity until the cyst is surgically removed. When surgery is delayed the cysts often develop infected tracts, which open up over the buttocks.

Treatment of the acute, infected pilonidal cyst consists of immediate incision of the inflamed cyst (after the injection of a very small amount of local anesthetic), in order that the pus will drain out of the cyst. This, of course, eases the pain immediately. I prefer, after incision and drainage of an acute pilonidal cyst, to place the patient on Keflex 250 mg. Q.I.D. until the inflammation subsides and then proceed with definitive surgery.

As soon as the acute infection is over the patient should be taken to surgery for the surgical removal of the cyst itself. For this, the patient is given a general anesthetic, and the cyst and all fistulous tracts are excised. The wound is then closed. The patient usually leaves the hospital on the first or second postoperative day.

PILONIDAL CYSTECTOMY

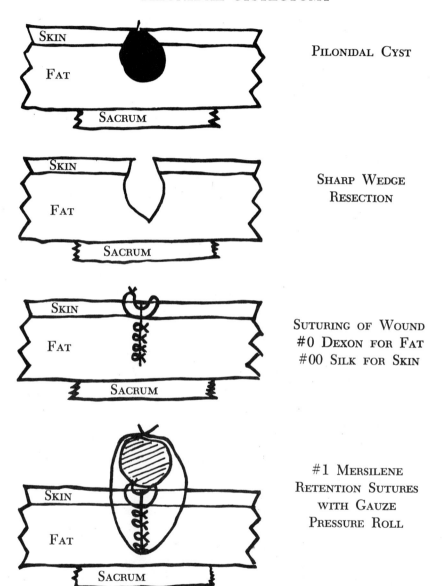

PILONIDAL CYST

SHARP WEDGE
RESECTION

SUTURING OF WOUND
#0 DEXON FOR FAT
#00 SILK FOR SKIN

#1 MERSILENE
RETENTION SUTURES
WITH GAUZE
PRESSURE ROLL

These patients will have a gauze dressing sewn to their skin to splint the wound and prevent the skin edges from pulling apart. After six or seven days this dressing is removed, as well as all other skin sutures. During the week after surgery it is mandatory that the dressing be kept dry.

Some pilonidal cysts are so very large that it is impossible to close the surgical wound completely. In these cases, the patient must come to the office once or twice weekly for dressing changes. It should be stated that the decision to close the surgical wound or leave it open is made at the surgical table according to the judgment of the surgeon. If at all possible, of course, the wound should be closed.

Pilonidal Cystectomy

The patient is placed in a left lateral Sims position and the surgical site painted with Mercresin. Sterile drapes are applied. 0.5cc of methyline blue is injected into the pilonidal orifice to aid in delineation of the cyst. An elliptical incision is made about the pilonidal cyst. The caudal end of the elliptical island is grasped with a Lahey thyroid tenaculum and Adair Allis forceps are used to grasp the remainder of the island skin. These are used for elevating the island to facilitate dissection. The pilonidal cyst and fistulous tract are excised by blunt and dull dissection, adhering closely to the cyst itself. The subcutaneous tissue is approximated with #0 Dexon suture. The skin edges are approximated with #00 silk suture.

Deep retention sutures of #1 Mersilene are placed in the mid-areas of the incision, and a large gauze dressing is sewn to the wound, creating a pressure dressing, splint, and reminder to the patient to limit his activity. The patient is instructed not to tamper with this dressing and not get it wet. All sutures are removed in seven to eight days, resulting in a satisfactory primary closure of the wound.

124